Keto Diet After 50

The Ultimate Ketogenic Diet Guide for People Over 50 to Lose Weight, Prevent Disease and Stay Healthy. Includes 100+ Easy to Follow Recipes and a 21-Day Meal Plan for Weight Loss

Vivian Cooper

Table of Contents

Table of Contents *3*

Introduction...*10*

Challenges For Over 50 11

Specifically for Women 11

Chapter 1: You & Keto *13*

Ketogenic Technique Levels..14

Scientific Ketogenic Benefits..14

Ketogenic 'Good' Fats 16

Ketogenic Dairy Selections 16

Ketogenic Homemade Cheese Options................................... 17

Almond Milk Pepper Jack..18

Baked Almond "Feta" 19

Cashew Cheddar Cheese 20

Swiss Cheese 21

Ketogenic Flour Options 22

Ketogenic Sweetener Options 22

Ketogenic Carbohydrate Balance 23

Ketogenic Protein Picks 23

Fish & Seafood 23

Poultry 24

Meat Choices 24

Ketogenic Iron Sources 24

Ketogenic Foods to Avoid or Eliminate 25

Chapter 2: Delicious Breakfast & Brunch Specialties *29*

Breakfast Custards 29

    Baked Custard - Dairy-Free 29

    Old-Fashioned Baked Custard - Heavy Cream 31

Egg Options 33

    Bacon & Egg Fat Bombs 33

    Best Scrambled Eggs 34

    Cream Cheese Eggs 35

    Ham & Egg Cups 36

    Ham & Spinach Mini Quiche 37

    Sausage Egg Casserole 38

    Scrambled Eggs with Mayo 39

Other Delicious Options 40

    Bacon & Brie Frittata 40

    BLT Brunch Wrap 42

    Blueberry Muffins 43

    Cauliflower & Cheddar Hash Browns 44

    Crispy Light Waffles 45

    Egg Muffins 47

    Flaxseed Porridge 48

    Hot Pockets 49

    Macadamia Keto Pancakes 50

    Pigs in Pancakes 51

    Sausage Gravy & Biscuits 53

Chapter 3: Luncheon Salad & Soup Specialties **54**

Salad Options 54

    Citrus Cauliflower Salad 54

    Rainbow Salad 56

    Snap Pea & Scallion Salad – Hot 57

Spinach - Broccoli - Feta Salad 58

Soup Options 59

Buffalo Chicken Soup 59

Cauliflower Beef Curry 61

Cauliflower & Kielbasa Soup 62

Chicken Zoodle Soup 63

Colby Cauliflower Soup & Pancetta Chips 64

Creamy Taco Soup 65

Italian Sausage Soup With Tomatoes & Zucchini Noodles 66

Shirataki Soup 68

Chapter 4: Lunchtime & Dinner Side Dish & Bread Specialties **69**

Avocado Tuna Melt Bites 69

Cabbage Patties 70

Cool & Spicy Jicama Slaw 71

Creamy Green Cabbage 72

Creamy Spinach-Rich Ballet 73

Dried Beef & Cream Cheese Ball 74

Garlic & Olive Oil Spaghetti Squash 75

Marinara Zoodles 76

Mushroom & Cauliflower Risotto 77

Red Pepper Zoodles 78

Stuffed Mushrooms 79

Zucchini Noodle Gratin 80

Flatbread Specialties 82

Buttery Low-Carb Flatbread 82

Indian Cuisine Naan Bread 83

Rosemary - Oregano & Thyme Flatbread 85

Chapter 5: Seafood Specialties **87**

    Crab Cakes 87

    Crunchy Fish and Chaffle Bites 88

    Mediterranean Grilled Ahi Tuna 89

    Parmesan Crusted Tilapia 90

    Parmesan Shrimp 91

    Salmon Cakes 93

    Shrimp Scampi 94

    Shrimp Scampi For Garlic Lovers 95

Chapter 6: Poultry Specialties **96**

    Balsamic Grilled Chicken Breast 96

    Chicken Nuggets 97

    Creamy Chicken Broccoli 99

    Fiesta Lime Chicken 100

    Parmesan Chicken 101

    Quick & Easy Creamy Mushroom Chicken 102

Chapter 7: Pork - Lamb & Beef Specialties **103**

  Pork Options 103

    Asian-Inspired Pork Chops 103

    Crockpot Pork Chops 104

    Hot Tex-Mex Pork Casserole 105

    Maple Country-Style Pork Ribs - Slow-Cooked 106

  Lamb Options 107

    Lamb & Asparagus with Tangy Sauce 107

    Kofta Kebab 108

    Roasted Leg of Lamb 109

  Beef Options 110

    Bacon Burger & Cabbage Stir Fry 110

BBQ Flank Steak 111

Cabbage Rolls - Slow Cooked 112

Creamy Burrito Bake 114

Mississippi Pot Roast 115

Nacho Skillet Steak 116

Skillet Cabbage Tacos 118

Chapter 8: Snacks & Appetizer Specialties 119

Smoothies 119

Avocado-Raspberry Smoothie.. 119

Blueberry Yogurt Smoothie 120

Cinnamon Smoothie.. 121

Strawberry Almond Smoothies 122

Delicious Snacks...123

Avocado & Bacon Caesar Deviled Eggs 123

Bacon-Wrapped Brussel Sprouts 125

Cheese Quesadilla 126

Cobb Salad Bacon Cups 127

Roasted Salt & Pepper Radish Chips............................128

Sweet Mustard Mini Sausages 129

Tasty Bacon & Cheese Balls 130

Zucchini Nacho Chips 131

Pizza Time 132

Cauliflower Pizza Crust 132

Crunchy Cheese Pizza with Mushrooms & Pepperoni.....134

Healthy Veggie Pizza on Flourless Cauliflower Crust.....135

Vegetarian Spinach Keto Flatbread...............................136

Chapter 9: Dessert Specialties.................................. 137

Pudding Favorites 137

Avocado & Chocolate Pudding 137

Cheesecake Pudding 138

Delicious Cakes 139

Carrot Almond Cake 139

Chocolate Lava Cake 140

Glazed Pound Cake 141

Lemon Cake 143

Spice Cakes 144

Vanilla - Sour Cream Cupcakes 145

Bar Cakes & Cookies 146

Browned Butter Chocolate Chip Blondies 146

Chocolate Chip Cookies 148

Key Lime Bars 149

Raspberry Fudge 151

Sunflower Seed Surprise Cookies 152

Pies & Cheesecakes 153

Keto Pie Crust 153

Delicious Cheesecake 154

Low-Carb Chocolate Cheesecake 156

Fat Bombs 157

Carrot Cake Fat Bombs 157

Pumpkin Spice Fat Bombs 159

Strawberry Ginger Fat Bomb 160

Chapter 10: Your 21-Day Meal Plan 161

Day 1: 16.7 Total Net Carbs 161

Day 2: 16.4 Total Net Carbs 161

Day 3: 18.16 Total Net Carbs 161

Day 4: 20.5 Total Net Carbs 162

Day 5: 14.39 Total Net Carbs 162

Day 6: 11.7 Total Net Carbs 162

Day 7: 14.5 Total Net Carbs 163

Day 8: 20.2 Total Net Carbs 163

Day 9: 16.5 Total Net Carbs 163

Day 10: 12.34 Total Net Carbs 163

Day 11: 19.1 Total Net Carbs 164

Day 12: 15.36 Total Net Carbs 164

Day 13: 13.9 Total Net Carbs 164

Day 14: 16.4 Total Net Carbs 165

Day 15: 21 Total Net Carbs 165

Day 16: 18.3 Total Net Carbs 165

Day 17: 19.16 Total Net Carbs 165

Day 18: 19 Total Net Carbs 166

Day 19: 15.64 Total Net Carbs 166

Day 20: 12 Total Net Carbs 166

Day 21: 12.6 Total Net Carbs 167

Chapter 11: A Final Word – Exercise **170**

Conclusion **175**

Skip Meals... 175

The 5:2 Technique 175

Introduction

Congratulations on purchasing the *Keto Diet After 50,* and thank you for doing so. As you grow older, your body changes. You will probably have problems losing the extra pounds even if you have a workout plan in gear. That is where keto comes into play.

The following chapters will discuss the techniques used for you to reach ketosis, how ketosis occurs, and how to maintain appropriate macros to sustain a healthier lifestyle without tons of extra work. You have many new recipes with the serving amounts and nutritional information provided.

There are several ways you can begin your ketogenic diet. You will want to start slowly. Choose a simple plan until your body can adjust. You can eliminate those high-carb dishes of pasta, desserts, and bread from your diet plan. Add healthier carbs such as sweet potatoes.

Choose a non-stressful way to begin the keto diet plan. Start by purging the refrigerator and the pantry. Restock both areas with the ketogenic food items that you will see listed in this book. Routinely, drink a large glass of water and keep track of your ketones. As you will see, the plan is very flexible, so you can decide which method will work best for you as you start the first few days of the rest of your life.

Before we start, I want to give you a little bonus, the "10 Tips To Organize Your Kitchen Space & Save". You can find it by opening this link from your computer:

https://bit.ly/2HpwEuA

So, let's begin your new path with the keto diet!

If you appreciate my book, make sure to leave a short review on Amazon, thank you very much!

Challenges For Over 50

Since the ketogenic diet is so restrictive, it may be hard for some individuals to maintain. The ketogenic diet may not be appropriate for all people. For example, it's not recommended for the following populations:

- Women who are pregnant or breastfeeding

- People who have liver or kidney failure

- Individuals who have alcohol or drug use disorders

- People with type 1 diabetes

- Those who have pancreatitis

- People who have disorders that affect fat metabolism

- Those who have certain deficiencies, including carnitine deficiency

- Individuals who have a blood disorder known as porphyria

- People who can't maintain adequate nutritional intake

Specifically for Women

- Weight loss plateaus — or even weight gain — are a typical stumbling block for women on keto. One way to fight back is to incorporate more fat or try periods of intermittent fasting.

- Restricting your carbs and calories too much on a keto diet can lead to out-of-balance hormones.

- Adjusting your eating habits along with your cycle, can keep your keto lifestyle and hormones more in-sync.

- Women who notice their energy is dragging should do carb cycling — "carb-up" once or twice a week with starchy vegetables.

- If emotional eating is thwarting your keto efforts, break habit loops by switching your routine in small ways.

- Ditching a deprivation mindset can help you reframe the narrative around your diet, enabling you to stick with it.

These are mere possibilities and many of which you will not experience as you grow older. Everyone is different, and keto is a workable tool to remedy issues as you age with grace! Let's see how to get started.

Chapter 1: You & Keto

These are the basic guidelines for daily carbohydrates to consider as you blaze the path on the ketogenic diet plan:

- *Ketogenic 0-20 Carbs* is the scale used by physicians during its testing for epilepsy. It maintains the lowest level of carbs related to a restrictive medical diet. The patient is restricted from 10 to 15 grams each day - to ensure the proper ketosis levels remain. As you see, it must have a doctor's approval to keep your body functional and healthy.

- *Moderate 20-50 carbs* are considered if you are obese, have diabetes, or metabolically deranged; you will want to remain within these limits. Your body can achieve a ketosis state that supplies the ketone bodies. This is the theory used to calculate your meal plan.

- *Liberal 50-100 carbs* are the best incentive if you're active and lean and are attempting to maintain your weight.

As you now see, it is vital to experiment and categorize where you fall on the scales before you make any changes. As with any new diet changes, you should seek your doctor's advice. You will soon realize the keto diet is flexible - yet strict. Each individual will lose weight differently, and other people may not have the same goals as you. For now, as a beginner, you will be using the second method.

Ketogenic Technique Levels

The *standard ketogenic diet* (SKD) comprises moderate proteins with high-fat content and maintains low carbs. The averages vary, but the ratio usually operates using 5% on carbs, 75% for high-fat, and 20% for your protein counts.

The *targeted keto diet*, which is also called TKD, will provide you with a technique to add carbs to the diet plan while working out or are more active.

The *cyclical ketogenic diet* (CKD) entails a restricted five-day keto diet plan followed by two high-carbohydrate days.

The *high-protein keto diet* is comparable to the standard keto plan (SKD) in all aspects, except you will consume more protein.

Scientific Ketogenic Benefits

Accelerated Fat Loss for Overweight & Obese Individuals: Weight Loss And Anti-Aging is improved long term according to a Harvard Study in 2018. Those who participate in the keto's intermittent fasting phase diet plan may exceed healthy figures when it comes to weight. It is imperative to use the keto diet plan to get started on the right path for weight loss.

Epileptic Seizures: For children, reductions in seizures have occurred for children who have used the keto diet. The therapeutic keto diet used for epilepsy often restricts the carbs to fewer than 15 grams of carbs daily to further escalate your ketone levels. Don't try to reach these levels unless you have the supervision of a medical professional.

Dravet Syndrome, a severe form of epilepsy, is marked by prolonged, uncontrollable, and frequent seizures. Currently, available medications don't improve symptoms in about 1/3 of the Dravet Syndrome patients. A clinical study used 13 children with the syndrome to stay on the ketogenic diet for more than one year to remain seizure-free. Over 50% of the group decreased in the frequency of the seizures. It was reported that six of the patients stopped the diet later, and one remains seizure-free.

Improvement of Your Cholesterol Profile: An arterial buildup is typically associated with triglyceride and cholesterol levels, proven to improve with the keto diet plan. Cut down your chance of heart disease. The triglycerides found in large amounts in carbohydrates are also found in high concentrations in those who have experienced cardiovascular problems.

Blood Pressure Levels Lowered: When you begin the ketogenic diet, your blood pressure may become lower, making you feel dizzy at first. Don't worry or feel overly concerned because that's a clear indication that the carbohydrates are working. However, suppose you are currently taking medications. It's a good idea to speak with your physician about the possibility of lowering some of your doses during the time that you are on the ketogenic plan.

Regulate Your Blood Sugar: According to a London 2005 Study, the ketogenic diet can help reduce the "bad" LDL cholesterol, inflammatory markers, blood triglycerides, and blood sugar for those with type 2 diabetes.

Polycystic Ovary Syndrome (PCOS) Improves: This is an endocrine disorder affecting young women of childbearing years. It is also associated with insulin resistance, obesity, and hyperinsulinemia. A 6-month study concluded a significant improvement in weight loss in fasting women over 24 weeks. The group limited carb intake to 20 grams daily for 24 weeks.

The ketogenic plan also helps other conditions, including Alzheimer' Disease, Parkinson's Disease, chronic inflammation, and migraines.

Ketogenic 'Good' Fats

You have many options to receive fats that will not have a 'bad' effect on your ketogenic diet. Select organic oil, including red palm oil, avocado, sesame, olive, and flaxseed oil. Also, select other fats, including unsalted butter, chicken fat, duck fat, and beef tallow.

Olive oil dates back for centuries to a time where oil was used for anointing kings and priests. It's a high-quality oil maintaining low-acidity, making this oil have a smoke point as high as 410° Fahrenheit. That's higher than most cooking applications call for, making olive oil more heat-stable than many other cooking fats. It contains zero carbs for two teaspoons.

Monounsaturated fats, such as in olive oil, are also linked with better blood sugar regulation, including lower fasting glucose and reducing inflammation throughout the body. Olive oil also helps to prevent cardiovascular disease. It protects your vascular system's integrity by lowering LDL, which is also called your 'bad' cholesterol. You can choose olives at one net carb for three jumbo - 5 large/10 small.

Purchase macadamia oil for its high smoke point of 390° Fahrenheit. It carries a mild flavor, which is a super alternative for olive oil in mayonnaise.

Ghee has zero carbs for one teaspoon. Unsweetened flaked coconut is only two net carbs for 3 tbsp.

Ketogenic Dairy Selections

Before beginning the keto way of life, you need to understand - dairy and dairy products are essential ketogenic components. If you're lactose intolerant, maybe the plan isn't for you. The amounts should be monitored to no more than four ounces daily.

Choose dairy products that have been cultured and are keto-friendly. The number one choice is unsweetened almond milk. Almond milk is calcium-fortified. An 8 ounce portion = 300-450 mg per 225 grams. You can also choose from hemp milk and flax milk.

Do you know the difference between butter and ghee? Butter consists of water, milk solids, and butterfat, whereas ghee, an Indian staple, includes pure butterfat. The ghee, or clarified butter as it's called, also contains medium-chain fatty acids that assist your immune system and digestion.

Grass-fed butter can promote fat loss, and butter is almost carb-free. The butter is a naturally occurring fatty acid that is rich in conjugated linoleic acid (CLA). It is suitable

Heavy whipping cream is used in many of your ketogenic recipes. It has only 5 grams of fat per tablespoon.

Ketogenic Homemade Cheese Options

There are quite a few packaged options for dairy-free cheese, but there are just as many recipes for homemade alternatives, from cheese balls to sauces. These are all keto- and vegan-friendly for your convenience. Here are a few different ones to get you started.

Almond Milk Pepper Jack

Ingredients:
- Onion powder (.33 tsp.)
- Almond milk (12 oz. - divided)
- Red pepper flakes (.33 tsp.)
- Chickpea flour (1 tbsp.)
- Agar powder (3 tsp.)
- Salt (.33 tsp.)
- Tapioca (2 tbsp.)
- Garlic powder (.33 tsp.)
- Apple cider vinegar (1 tsp.)
- Lemon juice (1 tsp.)
- Olive oil (2 tbsp.)
- Yeast (2 tbsp.)

Preparation Technique:
1. Prepare the container to be used as a mold by greasing it well.
2. Combine the starches in a large bowl and whisk well before adding the almond milk, chickpea flour, spices, salt, lemon juice, and olive oil.
3. Prepare a saucepan using the medium-temperature setting. Add the agar and 1 cup of milk. Let it cook for four minutes past the point it begins to boil - at which point you will want to turn the heat to low before adding in the starch as well as the almond milk.
4. Add the red pepper flakes and do a taste test for seasoning. You want to overcompensate the salt and spice because some of the flavors will be lost as it solidifies.
5. Increase the heat to medium before letting everything cook an additional five minutes, stirring regularly.
6. Transfer the pan to the countertop and add the pepper flakes. Empty the mixture into a greased container.
7. Chill for at least 1 hour, then grate into your recipe.

Baked Almond "Feta"

Ingredients:
- Salt (1 tsp.)
- Cloves of garlic (2 minced)
- Water (.5 cup)
- Lemon juice (.25 cup)
- Olive oil (2.5 tbsp.)
- Cheesecloth (3 pieces)

Preparation Technique:
1. Mince and add the garlic with the salt, olive oil, water, and lemon juice into a blender. Blend well until it is smooth and creamy.
2. Cover a small bowl using the cheesecloth before adding in the blended mixture.
3. Form the cheesecloth into a ball and secure the top.
4. Set the cheese ball into a strainer and place over the bowl. Let sit for 12 hours or overnight.
5. Ensure your oven is set to 180° Fahrenheit.
6. Add the mixture from the cheesecloth onto a baking dish that has been greased.
7. Bake for about 42 minutes. Cool and use as desired.

Cashew Cheddar Cheese

Ingredients:
- Raw cashews (.5 cup + 2 tbsp.)
- Powdered onion (1 tsp.)
- Sea salt (2 tsp.)
- Unsweetened soy milk (1.75 cups)
- Garlic powder (1 pinch)
- Yeast (.33 cup)
- Agar powder (8 tsp.)
- Lemon juice (1 tbsp.)
- Yellow or white miso (2 tbsp.)
- Canola oil (.25 cup)
- Optional: Truffle oil & chives
- Also Needed: Food processor

Preparation Technique:
1. Brush three or four small ramekins with oil.
2. Add the cashews to the processor. Pulse well. Add in the powdered onion, salt, garlic powder, and yeast to the processor. Pulse again until combined.
3. Add the agar, oil, and milk in a saucepan. Once the mixture boils, reduce the temperature to low-medium. Let it simmer, covered for 10 minutes. Stir as needed to ensure the agar is well dissolved.
4. Add the mixture to the food processor and work it steadily for 2 minutes until the mixture has combined. Blend in the miso, lemon juice, and any additional flavoring ingredients.
5. For sliced or grated cheese, cover the results and refrigerate for 4 hours until firm before removing the "cheese" from the ramekin using a sharp knife.
6. If it is melted cheese you're after, wait until the "cheese" has hardened and then melt by placing in a saucepan and heating using medium heat. Mix in additional soy milk to achieve your desired consistency.
7. If covered and refrigerated, the cheese will keep for 4 days.

Swiss Cheese

Ingredients:
- Powdered agar (1.66 tbsp.)
- Water (1.66 cups)
- Onion flakes (1 tbsp.)
- Yeast (.33 cup)
- Ground dill (.33 tbsp.)
- Soaked cashews (.66 cup)
- Salt (1 pinch)
- Tahini (2 tbsp.)
- Powdered garlic (.33 tbsp.)
- Lemon (1 juiced)
- Dijon mustard (2 tsp.)

Preparation Technique:
1. Oil and set aside a storage container, ramekin, or mold of your choice.
2. To the blender, add water, cashews, lemon juice, nutritional yeast, mustard, tahini, garlic, salt, onion flakes, dill, and garlic powder. Blend until the mixture is entirely smooth, occasionally stopping to test for grit. It usually takes anywhere from 1-3 minutes depending upon your blender.
3. In a saucepan, bring to boil 1 cup of water. Slowly add the agar while whisking. Let the pot simmer for 10 minutes, whisking as needed to ensure the agar dissolves completely. Add to the blender and mix until creamy.
4. Empty the finished mixture into an oiled container and let cool uncovered in the refrigerator.
5. When cooled, cover and chill for several hours.
6. To make the "Swiss holes," use a plastic straw and poke holes into the cheese on angles at random intervals.
7. Slice and enjoy on sandwiches, crackers, or any other delicious way you choose!

Ketogenic Flour Options

Transitioning into the ketogenic way of living can be made simpler by using low-carb substitutions for common goods used in cooking and baking. These are just a few ways keto-friendly products can be used to save the carbohydrates and provide you with an alternative plan.

Almond Flour: Almond flour is a suitable replacement and is used as all-purpose flour. Each one-quarter cup portion is only three carbohydrates per gram. Step one involves blanching the almonds. Toss them into boiling water to remove the skins. Next, you will grind the flour into a finely ground product that is an excellent choice for cakes, cookies, and pie crusts.

Sesame Flour: Finely grind sesame seeds to prepare the flour into a texture similar to wheat flour. Combine with psyllium flour for your baking needs to ensure the light texture of high-carb white bread.

Coconut Flour: You can use coconut flour in many of the keto diet meals. When using coconut flour, remember it isn't a 1:1 ratio. In comparison, you can substitute as little as 1/3 cup to 1/4 cup of coconut flour. Use one-part water to one-part coconut flour and whisk together to use as a thickening agent. Add it to hot liquids such as soup. It's high in fiber - making it super absorbent. You can add oils, eggs, and other fluids as needed. Use the coconut flour at times when you are sautéing or frying foods.

Ketogenic Sweetener Options

Stevia Drops offer flavors, including English toffee, hazelnut, vanilla, and chocolate. You can make sweetened coffee or drinks quickly. However, everyone is different, and some think the drops are bitter to taste. Therefore, only use three drops to equal one teaspoon of sugar.

Swerve Granular Sweetener is also an excellent choice as a blend made from non-digestible carbs sourced from starchy root veggies and select fruits. It is a perfect choice for those who do not like the taste of stevia.

Swerve is on the market as a one-to-one substitute. However, start with ¾ of a teaspoon for every one of sugar. Increase the portion as desired. Swerve also has confectioners/powdered sugar for your baking needs. On the downside, it is more expensive than other products such as the Pyure.

Ketogenic Carbohydrate Balance

Research has indicated that "unlike other low-carb diets, which focus on protein, a keto plan centers on fat, which supplies as much as 90% of your daily calories." Since there's no set rule for carb intake, you will want to be sure you are consuming the right amounts of food to keep your diet balanced for ketosis. You will be gradually working your way through the plan by consuming plenty of vegetables, minimal intake of carbs, and two to three fruit pieces daily.

Ketogenic Protein Picks

Protein can help slow down your digestion process, helping you feel satisfied with your food consumption. It works as a fat-burner and aids in muscle repair and growth. You will be using many of these choices in your meal plan.

Fish & Seafood

Include wild-caught fish, including tuna, trout, salmon, snapper, catfish, flounder, cod, halibut, mahi-mahi, or mackerel. Enjoy shellfish such as crabs, clams, lobster, oysters, scallops, squid, shrimp, or mussels.

Poultry

Choose from duck, pheasant, or quail. Select chicken breasts, thighs, drumsticks, or ground options. Serve ground turkey and breast portions.

Shop for a local area market for free-range egg options. You can scramble, fry, boil, or devil eggs for a picnic or any occasion.

Meat Choices

Grass-fed options are preferred because it has a better fatty acid count. Choose from lamb, veal, goat, or other wild game. Cuts of beef include flank steak, sirloin, chuck roast, and lean ground beef. Choose pork including, chops, loins, and ham (no added sugar). If you know a hunter, deer venison is a healthy choice.

Ketogenic Iron Sources

- Coconut milk: 3.3 mg for each 3.5 oz./100 g

- Pumpkin seeds: 4.2 mg for each 1 oz./28 g

- Chia seeds: 2.2 mg for each 1 oz./28 g

- Sesame seeds: 4.1 mg for each 1 oz./28 g

- White mushrooms - cooked: 2.7 mg for each 3.5 oz./100 g

- Spinach - cooked: 3.6 mg for each 3.5 oz./100 g

- Dark chocolate: 3.3 mg for each 1 oz./28 g

Ketogenic Foods to Avoid or Eliminate

The foods listed in this segment may be used in some of your ketogenic recipes, but generally in small amounts. These are guidelines, so you'll better understand how quickly carbs add up when you begin preparing your meals.

You need to be aware of the ones that fall into this category:

- *Processed Polyunsaturated Fats:* Avoid these oils: Sunflower, peanut, grapeseed, sesame, corn, canola, and soybean.

- *Processed Trans Fats:* Avoid fast foods, processed foods, margarine, and commercially prepared baked goods.

Milk

Keto dieters should avoid milk that contains moderate or excessive amounts of carbs. Here are several types of milk that you should avoid while on keto with the net carbs listed for one cup:

- Cow's milk (12 grams): Cow's milk contains lactose - milk sugar. This includes evaporated milk, ultra-filtered milk, and raw cow's milk.

- Oat milk (17 grams): Oat milk is made from oats, which are naturally high in carbs. This makes oat milk inappropriate for keto.

- Goat's milk (11 grams): This is another bad choice with its natural sugars, making it too high in carbs to be keto-friendly.

- Rice milk (21 grams) is naturally high in carbs.

Grains to Avoid:

First, you need to realize grains are made from carbohydrates. This list is based on one cup servings. Avoid bread, pasta, pizza crusts, or crackers and cookies made with these grains:

- Buckwheat: 33 carbs - 6 protein - 1 gram fat

- Wheat: (1 slice wheat bread) 14 carbs - 3 protein - 1 gram fat

- Barley: 44 carbs - 4 protein - 1 gram fat

- Quinoa: 39 carbs - 8 protein - 4 grams fat

- Corn: 32 carbs - 4 protein - 1 gram fat

- Millet: 41 carbs - 6 protein - 2 grams fat

- Bulgur: 33 carbs - 5.6 protein - 0.4 grams fat

- Amaranth: 46 carbs - 9 protein - 4 grams fat

- Oats: 36 carbs - 6 protein - 3 grams fat

- Rice: 45 carbs - 5 protein - 2 grams fat

- Rye: 15 carbs - 3 protein - 1 gram fat

Sugars to Avoid:

- Raw Sugar: 12 grams of carbs - 0 protein - 0 grams fat

- Agave Nectar: 14 grams of carbs - 0 protein - 0 grams fat

- Honey: 17 grams of carbs - 0 protein -0 grams fat

- Maple Syrup: 14 grams of carbs - 0 protein - 0 grams fat

- Cane Sugar: 12 grams of carbs - 0 protein - 0 grams fat

- High-fructose Corn Syrup: 14 grams of carbs - 0 protein - 0 grams fat

- Turbinado Sugar: 12 carbs - 0 protein - 0 grams fat

Peanut Butter

Try natural peanut butter, but use caution because they contain high carbohydrates and Omega-6s. Macadamia nut butter is a wise alternative.

Bacon & Sausage

Avoid bacon and sausage that has extra fillers or has been cured in sugar.

Processed Foods

If you see carrageenan on the label, it's best to leave it on the shelf. Don't feel too guilty if you crave all of those processed foods. It happens. As a rule of thumb, look for labels with the least amount of ingredients. Usually, the ones that provide the most nutrition are listed in those shorter lists.
These are just a few examples of processed snacks to avoid while on a ketogenic diet. Some are surprising because they were deemed for years as a healthy and nutritious snack.

- Cereal Bars

- Crackers

- Rice cakes

- Popcorn

- Flavored Nuts

- Pretzels

- Potato Chips

- Protein Bars

Do you recognize any of them?

Let's see how it works using the ketogenic recipes!

Chapter 2: Delicious Breakfast & Brunch Specialties

Breakfast Custards

Baked Custard - Dairy-Free

Servings Provided: 6
Prep & Cook Time: 1 hour 20 minutes
Macro Counts - Per Serving:
- Calories: 246
- Net Carbohydrates: 3 g
- Protein: 6 g
- Fat Content: 24 g

Ingredients:
- Unsweetened - full-fat coconut milk (3 cups/678 g)
- Raw eggs (4 large/200 g)
- Pure vanilla extract (1 tsp./2.5 g) or scrapings from ½ of a vanilla pod
- Optional Sprinkle Topping: Nutmeg/cinnamon
  Also Needed:
- Glass baking dish - to hold serving containers
- 6 oz. glass custard/serving dishes

Preparation Technique:
1. Warm the oven to 350 °Fahrenheit.
2. Boil enough water to come ½ inch from the top of the outside of the custard cups. Place the cups into the pan. (Wait to fill the dish with water.)
3. Whisk the eggs with the milk, sweetener, and vanilla and add it to the cups. Sprinkle cinnamon/nutmeg over the top as desired.

4. Arrange the holding tray on the oven rack and pour the hot water to make the water bath. Bake the custard for 45 minutes.
5. Check for doneness. Insert a knife into the middle of the cup. It's ready if it comes out without custard attached.
6. Carefully transfer the dishes to the countertop or serving tray to serve. Add any leftovers to the fridge with a covering of foil or plastic wrap.

Old-Fashioned Baked Custard - Heavy Cream

Servings Provided: 6
Prep & Cook Time: 1 hour 20 minutes
Macro Counts - Per Serving:
- Calories: 370
- Net Carbohydrates: 3 g
- Protein: 6 g
- Fat Content: 37 g

Ingredients:
- Water (.5 cup)
- 36% heavy cream (2.5 cups/565 g)
- Raw egg (4 large/200 g)
- Pure vanilla extract (1 tsp./2.5 g) or Pod scrapings (½ of a vanilla pod)
  Optional Toppings:
- Sweetener - your preference
- Nutmeg or cinnamon
  Also Needed:
- Glass baking dish
- Glass custard dishes (6 oz.)

Preparation Technique:
1. Measure and boil water to make a water bath using the baking dish. It needs to be enough to extend three-quarters of the way up the custard cups (fill in the last step).
2. Set the oven at 350° Fahrenheit.
3. Use a mixing container to whisk the eggs with the water, vanilla, cream, and sweetener - if using.
4. Scoop the custard into the serving cups. (Place the cups in the baking dish before you begin.) Sprinkle using a dusting of the nutmeg or cinnamon to your liking.
5. Arrange the baking dish on the oven rack. Pour the hot water into the ½-inch marker of the cups.

6. Set a timer to bake for 45 minutes. It should be firmly set. Test it using a knife in the middle of the custard. If it comes out mostly clean, it's ready.
7. Serve the custard warm. Store it with a covering of foil or plastic in the refrigerator.

Egg Options

Bacon & Egg Fat Bombs

Servings Provided: 6
Prep & Cook Time: 55 minutes
Macro Counts - Per Serving:
- Calories: 185
- Net Carbohydrates: 0.2 g
- Protein: 5 g
- Fat Content: 18 g

Ingredients:
- Bacon slices (4.2 oz. or 4 large)
- Large organic eggs (2)
- Ghee or butter (.25 cup)
- Black pepper (1 pinch)
- Salt (.25 tsp.)
- Mayonnaise (2 tbsp.)

Preparation Technique:
1. Set the oven temperature at 375⁰ Fahrenheit.
2. Arrange the bacon slices on a parchment paper-lined baking tin. Bake it;/ for 10 to 15 minutes. Drain and reserve the grease.
3. On the stovetop, boil the eggs for ten minutes in salted water. Quickly add them into an ice bath to cool. Peel and slice the eggs and add the butter or ghee to the eggs. Smash with a fork.
4. Combine the pepper, salt, mayonnaise, and bacon grease. Stir thoroughly and place it in the refrigerator for 20-30 minutes.
5. Meanwhile, crumble the strips of bacon in a container for breading the bombs. Form six balls using an ice cream scoop for uniform sizing. Roll them in the bits and place them in the fridge.

Best Scrambled Eggs

Servings Provided: 2
Prep & Cook Time: 10 minutes
Macro Counts - Per Serving:
- Calories: 161.5
- Net Carbohydrates: 2.9 g
- Protein: 13.7 g
- Fat Content: 10.1 g

Ingredients:
- Eggs (4 large)
- Salt and pepper (as desired)
- Skim or 1% milk (.25 cup)
- Fresh parsley (2 tbsp.)
- Cooking oil spray (as needed)

Preparation Technique:
1. Finely chop the parsley. Break eggs into a bowl and add the milk, pepper, salt, and parsley. Whisk until thoroughly combined.
2. Warm a skillet using the med-high temperature setting and lightly spritz it using the cooking spray.
3. Pour eggs into the pan, pushing them around the pan with a non-metal spatula until the eggs are set and no liquid remains (5 min.).
4. Scrape the pan and continue stirring to keep the eggs light and fluffy.
5. Note: For the best results, don't use egg beaters! They will not properly cook.

Cream Cheese Eggs

Servings Provided: 1
Prep & Cook Time: 7-10 minutes
Macro Counts - Per Serving:
- Calories: 341
- Net Carbohydrates: 3 g
- Protein: 15 g
- Fat Content: 29 g

Ingredients:
- Butter (1 tbsp.)
- Eggs (2)
- Soft cream cheese with chives (2 tbsp.)

Preparation Technique:
1. Heat a skillet and melt the butter. Whisk the eggs with the cream cheese.
2. Add to the pan and serve when ready.

Ham & Egg Cups

Servings Provided: 9
Prep & Cook Time: 25 minutes
Macro Counts - Per Serving:
- Calories: 117
- Net Carbohydrates: 0.96 g
- Protein: 7.72 g
- Fat Content: 9.17 g

Ingredients:
- Fresh eggs, fresh (5 large/250 grams)
- 36% heavy cream (.5 cup/135 grams)
- Natural Uncured Black Forest Ham by Applegate (7 oz. pkg.)
- Coconut oil (5 grams/1 tsp.)
- Also Needed: Muffin tin (at least 9-count)

Preparation Technique:
1. Set the oven temperature at 425° Fahrenheit. Lightly grease nine wells/cups of a muffin tin with a spritz of cooking oil.
2. Arrange one slice of ham in each of the muffin wells/cups, pressing the slices of ham into the cups centered with the ham covering the sides and bottoms.
3. Whisk and thoroughly combine the cream, egg, pepper, and salt. Fill nine of the muffin cups.
4. Bake until the egg centers have puffed, and the eggs are totally set (7-10 min). They might slightly jiggle - if shaken but shouldn't be runny/liquid.
5. Add desired garnishes such a green onion or roasted red peppers, or feta cheese, but add the extra carbs.

Ham & Spinach Mini Quiche

Servings Provided: 2
Prep & Cook Time: 20 minutes
Macro Counts - Per Serving:
- Calories: 210
- Net Carbohydrates: 2 g
- Protein: 20 g
- Fat Content: 13 g

Ingredients:
- Chopped spinach (.75 cup)
- Chopped leek (.25 cup)
- Whisked eggs (3)
- Diced ham (4 slices)
- Coconut milk (.25 cup)
- Baking powder (.5 tsp.)
- Pepper & salt (to taste)
- Also Needed: 4 small quiche or tart pans

Preparation Technique:
1. Set the oven temperature to reach 350° Fahrenheit.
2. Combine all of the fixings in a large mixing container.
3. Empty the mixture into the pans.
4. Bake for 15 minutes. Serve or store for later.

Sausage Egg Casserole

Servings Provided: 12
Prep & Cook Time: 30 minutes
Macro Counts - Per Serving:
- Calories: 200.5
- Net Carbohydrates: 2.1 g
- Protein: 15.7 g
- Fat Content: 39.4 g

Ingredients:
- Cooked - browned breakfast sausage - low-fat & reduced-sodium (12 oz.)
- Eggs (12 large)
- Skim milk (.25 cup)
- Low-fat cheddar cheese (2 cups - shredded)
- Black pepper (.25 tsp.)

Preparation Technique:
1. Set the oven to 375° Fahrenheit. Use paper or lightly grease a 12-count muffin pan or grease a casserole dish.
2. Add the batter and bake for ½ hour. Cool for five minutes before serving.

Scrambled Eggs with Mayo

Servings Provided: 1
Prep & Cook Time: 15 minutes
Macro Counts - Per Serving:
- Calories: 307
- Net Carbohydrates: 0.99 g
- Protein: 6.6 g
- Fat Content: 30.81 g

Ingredients:
- Large raw egg (1 @ 50 g)
- Butter (10g)
- Organic mayonnaise - ex. - Trader Joe's (23 g)
- Salt (1 pinch)

Preparation Technique:
1. Prepare a small pan to melt the butter.
2. Whisk the mayo with the egg until thoroughly mixed.
3. Cook and swirl the egg until done. Serve promptly.

Other Delicious Options

Bacon & Brie Frittata

Servings Provided: 6
Prep & Cook Time: 30 minutes
Macro Counts - Per Serving:
- Calories: 338
- Net Carbohydrates: 1.7 g
- Protein: 18 g
- Fat Content: 27 g

Ingredients:
- Slices of bacon (8)
- Eggs (8 large)
- Heavy whipping cream (.5 cup)
- Garlic (2 cloves)
- Salt and black pepper (.5 tsp. each)
- Brie sliced thin (easiest to do when it's cold (4 oz.)
- Also Needed: 10-inch oven-proof skillet

Preparation Technique:
1. Chop and fry the bacon in the skillet using the medium heat temperature setting until it is crispy. Transfer it to drain on a paper towel-lined plate. (Leave at least two to three tablespoons of bacon grease in the skillet and remove from heat). Let the skillet cool.
2. Mince the garlic. Whisk the eggs with the garlic, salt, pepper, cream, and about ⅔ of the cooked bacon. Set the

skillet over medium-low heat and swirl the remaining bacon grease to coat its bottom and sides.

3. Add the mix to the skillet (undisturbed) and cook for seven to ten minutes, leaving it somewhat loose to add the brie and rest of the bacon.

4. Warm the broiler and place the skillet on the second-highest rack.

5. Broil for about two to five minutes. Remove the pan and cool it for a couple of minutes to serve.

BLT Brunch Wrap

Servings Provided: 1
Prep & Cook Time: 10-15 minutes
Macro Counts - Per Serving:
- Calories: 256
- Net Carbohydrates: 2 g
- Protein: 8 g
- Fat Content: 24 g

Ingredients:
- Romaine or Iceberg lettuce leaves (2)
- Crispy fried bacon slices (4)
- Chopped tomatoes (.25 cup)
- Mayo (1 tbsp.)
- Optional: Pepper

Preparation Technique:
1. Rinse the leaves of lettuce and let them drain in a colander.
2. Prepare the bacon in a skillet or the microwave until it's crispy.
3. Spread a layer of mayonnaise on one side of the lettuce.
4. Chop and add the tomatoes and bacon bits. Season the wrap as desired.
5. Roll it up and serve.

Blueberry Muffins

Servings Provided: 12
Prep & Cook Time: 55 minutes
Macro Counts - Per Serving:
- Calories: 221
- Net Carbohydrates: 5 g
- Protein: 6 g
- Fat Content: 20 g

Ingredients:
- Almond flour (2 cups/224 g)
- Coconut flour (.25 cup (30 g)
- Konjac root fiber (2 tsp./8 g)
- Baking soda (4 g/1 tsp.)
- Salt (1 pinch)
- Baking powder (4 g/1 tsp.)
- Olive oil (.5 cup/108 g)
- Fresh eggs (3 large/150 g)
- Water (2-4 tbsp.)
- Fresh blueberries (.5 cup/74 g)

Preparation Technique:
1. Set the oven temperature at 350° Fahrenheit. Cover the muffin tin with 12 paper/foil liners.
2. Whisk/sift the almond flour with the coconut flour, baking powder, konjac root fiber, baking soda, and salt.
3. Mix in the eggs with the olive oil and two tablespoons of water into the dry components. Thoroughly whisk to combine (as the consistency of thick pancake batter).
4. Gently fold in the blueberries (about half to two-thirds full).
5. Bake the muffins until a toothpick inserted into the center remains clean when removed (35-40 min.).

Cauliflower & Cheddar Hash Browns

Servings Provided: 12 hash browns
Prep & Cook Time: 30 minutes
Macro Counts - Per Serving:
- Calories: 124
- Net Carbohydrates: 2.5 g
- Protein: 5 g
- Fat Content: 11 g

Ingredients:
- Frozen cauliflower rice - thawed (12 oz. bag)
- Arrowroot starch (15 grams/2 tbsp.)
- Optional: Black pepper, salt, onion powder, garlic powder & other seasonings
- Shredded cheddar cheese (226 grams/8 oz. bag)
- Avocado oil (46 grams or 1/3 cup)
- Also Needed: Waffle maker

Preparation Technique:
1. Warm a non-stick waffle maker while you prepare the hash brown mixture.
2. Remove most of the liquid from the cauliflower bag by using a knife's tip to poke a tiny hole. Thoroughly squeeze the bag and toss the rice with the seasonings and arrowroot starch in a mixing container.
3. Drizzle in the oil and shredded cheese, tossing to combine.
4. Portion the hash browns into the well's center (leaving the mix piled). Lower the lid to flatten the mixture. Cook until they are a deep golden brown. When done, the cheese will be crispy, making it easy to pop out of the waffle iron.
   Alternative Cooking Methods:
5. Option 1: You can also use a generously greased muffin tin in a 475 °Fahrenheit oven until crispy on the outside edges (10 min.).
6. Option 2: Prepare a non-stick skillet using the med-high temperature setting. Shape the portions into thick patties and fry on each side until crispy and golden brown.

**Crispy Light Waffles**

Servings Provided: 8
Prep & Cook Time: 25 minutes
Macro Counts - Per Serving:
- Calories: 140
- Net Carbohydrates: 1 g
- Protein: 4 g
- Fat Content: 11 g

Ingredients:
- Almond flour (.66 cup)
- Xanthan gum (1 tsp.)
- Coconut flour (.25 cup)
- Psyllium husk (1 tbsp.)
- Water (1 cup)
- Coconut oil/butter (.25 cup)
- Xylitol/swerve (3 tbsp.)
- Kosher salt (.25 tsp.)
- Eggs (3)
- Vanilla extract (1 tsp.)
- Baking powder (1.5 tsp.)
- Also Needed: Waffle Iron & Dutch oven

Preparation Technique:
1. Combine the coconut flour, xanthan gum, almond flour, and psyllium husk.
2. In a dutch oven, warm the water, sweetener, butter, and salt until it simmers. Adjust the temperature setting and whisk in the flour mixture. Stir until it forms a ball or about one to three minutes.
3. Arrange the dough in the bowl to cool for five minutes. You want the dough to be warm, not hot.
4. Lightly whisk the eggs - adding one egg at a time. Blend with an electric mixer. Stir in the baking powder and

vanilla extract. It should form an elastic-type dough. Let the dough rest for about ten minutes.

5. Heat the waffle iron using the high-temperature setting. Lightly grease the iron and spoon in the batter. Close the iron (8-12 min.) until golden.

6. The dough is suitable for a day or two in the fridge. The waffles are good for three days at room temperature.

Egg Muffins

Servings Provided: 12
Prep & Cook Time: 35 minutes
Macro Counts - Per Serving:
- Calories: 147
- Net Carbohydrates: 1 g
- Fat Content: 11 g
- Protein: 10 g

Ingredients:
- Eggs (12)
- Italian sausage (.5 lb.)
- 36% heavy cream (.25 cup)
- Garlic powder (.5 tsp.)
- Chives (2 tsp.)
- Himalayan pink salt (1-2 pinches)
- Also Needed: 12-count muffin tin

Preparation Technique:
1. Warm the oven to reach 350 °Fahrenheit.
2. Brown the sausage until thoroughly browned and cooked. Cool the meat in the pan, but do *not* drain off the fat.
3. Break the eggs into a large mixing container and add the cream. Mix and thoroughly whisk in the seasonings and any optional add-ins.
4. Fold in the meat and thoroughly mix it. Scoop it into a dozen well-greased muffin wells.
5. Bake for ½ hour or until the egg centers are set.

Flaxseed Porridge

Servings Provided: 1
Prep & Cook Time: 5 minutes
Macro Counts - Per Serving:
- Net Carbohydrates: 4 g
- Protein: 6 g
- Fat Content: 40 g

Ingredients:
- Flaxseed - plain or roasted is nutty-like (3 tbsp.)
- Coconut Milk - unsweetened (.5 cup)
- Butter (2.5 tsp.)
- Grapeseed oil (2 tsp.)
- Wild/frozen blueberries - ex. - Trader Joe's (2 tbsp.)
- Cinnamon (0.125 tsp.)

Preparation Technique:
1. Whisk the milk with the flaxseed in a microwave-safe bowl. Use one that will hold at least two cups of liquid. Cook until the mixture starts rising (30-45 sec.).
2. Transfer the container to the countertop and wait for it to cool for one minute.
3. Mix in the butter, oil, blueberries, and cinnamon. Stir thoroughly to coat the blueberries. Don't over-stir; it will make the porridge gummy.
4. *Note:* You can also make it using a small saucepan on the stovetop. You will remove the pan from the burner once the mixture starts to boil.

Hot Pockets

Servings Provided: 2
Prep & Cook Time: 35 minutes
Macro Counts - Per Serving:
- Calories: 287
- Net Carbohydrates: 2 g
- Protein: 24 g
- Fat Content: 25 g

Ingredients:
- Mozzarella cheese (.75 cup)
- Almond flour (.33 cup)
- Cooked bacon (3 slices)
- Unsalted butter (2 tbsp.
- Eggs (2)

Preparation Technique:
1. Warm the oven to reach 400° Fahrenheit.
2. Melt the cheese and combine with the flour. Roll out the dough between two layers of parchment baking paper.
3. Cook the bacon until crispy and set aside.
4. Heat a skillet and add the butter. When melted, whisk and pour in the eggs. Scramble until done. Roll the eggs and bacon on top of the dough to seal.
5. Bake them for 20 minutes until firm when touched and golden brown.

Macadamia Keto Pancakes

Servings Provided: 4
Prep & Cook Time: 20 minutes
Macro Counts - Per Serving:
- Calories: 300
- Net Carbohydrates: 1.5 g
- Fat Content: 30 g
- Protein: 6 g

Ingredients:
- Macadamia nuts – roasted (30 g)
- Raw egg (28 g)
- Optional: Vanilla Extract (3 drops)
- Pecan/macadamia nut oil (6 g)

Preparation Technique:
1. Finely chop the nuts in a blender.
2. Thoroughly whisk the egg, add it to the oil, and into the nuts.
3. Add vanilla if desired.
4. Lightly spritz a skillet using a baking oil spray.
5. Drop the batter into desired size circles and cook until nicely browned to serve.

Pigs in Pancakes

Servings Provided: 10 pancakes
Prep & Cook Time: 25-30 minutes
Macro Counts - Per Serving:
- Calories: 213
- Net Carbohydrates: 3.04 g
- Protein: 12.7 g
- Fat Content: 16.2 g

Ingredients:
- Almond flour - super-fine (1 cup)
- Coconut flour (.25 cup)
- Swerve sweetener (3 tbsp.)
- Salt (.25 tsp.)
- Baking powder (2 tsp.)
- Large eggs (4)
- Almond milk - unsweetened (.66 cup)
- Avocado oil/butter/ghee (.25 cup - melted)
- Vanilla extract (.5 tsp.)
- Butter or oil for a pan
- Breakfast sausages (10)
- For the Pan: Oil or butter as needed

Preparation Technique:
1. First, cook and cool the sausage.
2. Warm the oven to reach 300° Fahrenheit. Prepare a cookie sheet with a baking rack inside.
3. Whisk both types of flour with the swerve, salt, and baking powder. Whisk and add in the eggs, melted butter, milk, and vanilla extract until it's thoroughly combined.
4. Warm a skillet with butter using the medium temperature setting.
5. Use about two tablespoons of batter to create a thin line as long as your breakfast sausages (it will spread slightly as it heats). Place the cooked sausage in the middle and cover it with another tablespoon or so of batter. Continue to fill the

pan and cook them for two to three minutes on the first
side.

6. Carefully flip it over and continue cooking for another two
to three minutes. Transfer them to the prepared baking
rack and bake them for 10-15 minutes.

7. Note: Bob's Red Mill provides a high-quality flour for this
recipe.

Sausage Gravy & Biscuits

Servings Provided: 2
Prep & Cook Time: 40 minutes
Macro Counts - Per Serving:
- Calories: 425
- Net Carbohydrates: 2 g
- Protein: 22 g
- Fat Content: 36 g

Ingredients:
- Salt (.25 tsp.)
- Almond flour (.25 cup)
- Baking powder (.5 tsp.)
- Large egg white (1)
- Crumbled breakfast sausage (6 oz. pkg.)
- Chicken broth (.25 cup)
- Cream cheese (.25 cup)
- Pepper and salt (as desired)

Preparation Technique:
1. Warm the oven to reach 400º Fahrenheit. Prepare a baking tin with a sheet of parchment baking paper.
2. Whisk the salt, almond flour, and baking powder.
3. In another dish, whisk the egg whites to form stiff peaks.
4. Dice the butter into small pieces. Form a crumbled mixture in the dry components using the butter. Gently blend the butter into the egg whites.
5. Split the mixture into two portions on the paper-lined pan.
6. Bake them for 11 to 15 minutes.
7. Using the medium heat setting to warm the sausage. When browned, add the cream cheese, chicken broth, pepper, and salt.
8. Serve with the biscuits and a serving of the delicious gravy.
9. Prep time is just 15 minutes with a cooking time of only 25 minutes. What a treat in such a little amount of time!

Chapter 3: Luncheon Salad & Soup Specialties

Salad Options

Citrus Cauliflower Salad

Servings Provided: 4
Prep & Cook Time: 12-15 minutes
Macro Counts - Per Serving:
- Calories: 177
- Net Carbohydrates: 1 g
- Protein: 2 g
- Fat Content: 7 g

Ingredients:
  The Salad:
- Small Romanesco cauliflower (1 - divided)
- Seedless oranges (2)
- Broccoli (1 lb.)
  The Vinaigrette:
- Anchovies (4)
- Orange - juice & zest (1)
- Salted – unrinsed capers (1 tbsp.)
- Hot pepper (1)
- Salt and black pepper (as desired)
- E-V olive oil (4 tbsp._
- Also Needed: Instant Pot Cooker

Preparation Technique:
1. Slice the cauliflower into florets. Remove the peel and thinly slice the oranges. Finely chop the anchovies, capers, and hot peppers for the vinaigrette.
2. Prepare the vinaigrette fixings in a jar with a lid. Shake well and set aside.

3. Set up the Instant Pot with one cup of water and the steamer basket. Add the cauliflower to the basket and secure the lid. Set the timer for 6 minutes using low pressure. Quick-release the steam pressure when you hear the buzzer.
4. Transfer the florets to a serving dish with the prepared oranges. Toss.
5. Drizzle with the vinaigrette and enjoy.

Rainbow Salad

Servings Provided: 8
Prep & Cook Time: 5-6 minutes
Macro Counts - Per Serving:
- Calories: 109
- Net Carbohydrates: 1 g
- Protein: 15 g
- Fat Content: 9 g

Ingredients:
  The Dressing:
- Garlic cloves (2)
- Parsley (.25 cup)
- White balsamic vinegar (.5 cup)
- Olive oil (2 tbsp.)
- Salt & pepper (1 pinch)
  The Salad:
- Red cabbage (2 cups)
- Assorted salad greens (8 cups)
- Carrots (1 cup)
- Cucumber (1 cup)
- Raw sunflower seeds (.5 cup)
- Red & yellow bell pepper (1 each)

Preparation Technique:
1. Do the prep and measure all the fixings.
2. Mince the garlic and parsley. Chop the peppers, cabbage, and cucumber. Slice the carrots.
3. Whisk all of the dressing fixings in a mixing container. Pour into a serving container.
4. Drain the chickpeas and prep the veggies.
5. Prepare the salads and serve.

Snap Pea & Scallion Salad – Hot

Servings Provided: 1
Prep & Cook Time: 10 minutes + chill time
Macro Counts - Per Serving:
- Net Carbohydrates: 3 g
- Protein: 2 g
- Fat Content: 14 g

Ingredients:
- Sugar snap peas (50 g)
- Scallions - green & white parts (10 g)
- Sesame oil (2 g)
- Coconut aminos/or another keto-friendly soy sauce (2 g)
- Cider vinegar (3 g)
- Olive oil (11 g)
- Garlic powder (0.1 g)
- Sesame seeds (2 g)
- Optional Ingredient: Red chili flakes

Preparation Technique:
1. Slice the snap peas and diagonally slice the scallions.
2. Combine the sliced veggies with the rest of the fixings, tossing thoroughly to combine.
3. Cover with plastic wrap and place the container in the fridge for at least two hours.
4. Serve with a choice of protein, such as grilled chicken, shrimp, or salmon.

Spinach - Broccoli - Feta Salad

Servings Provided: 4
Prep & Cook Time: 15 minutes
Macro Counts - Per Serving:
- Calories: 397
- Net Carbohydrates: 4.9 g
- Fat Content: 3.8 g
- Protein: 9 g

Ingredients:
- Vinegar - white wine (1 tbsp.)
- Olive oil (2 tbsp.)
- Broccoli slaw (2 cups)
- Poppy seeds (2 tbsp.)
- Spinach (2 cups)
- Black pepper & salt (as desired)
- Walnuts (.33 cup)
- Sunflower seeds (.33 cup)
- Blueberries (.33 cup)
- Feta cheese (.66 cup crumbled)

Preparation Technique:
1. Chop the spinach and nuts.
2. Combine the slaw, spinach, blueberries, sunflower seeds, walnuts, and cheese.
3. Make the dressing (vinegar, oil, salt, pepper, and poppy seeds) and add to the salad.
4. Toss it and serve.

Soup Options

Buffalo Chicken Soup

Servings Provided: 6
Prep & Cook Time: 40 minutes
Macro Counts - Per Serving:
- Calories: 335
- Net Carbohydrates: 4 g
- Protein: 33 g
- Fat Content: 17 g

Ingredients:
- Olive oil (1 tbsp.)
- Medium onion (1)
- Garlic powder (1 tsp.)
- Chopped celery (2 cups)
- Dried thyme (1 tsp.)
- Chicken breasts (4)
- Hot sauce - ex. - Frank's Red (.25 cup/as desired)
- Chicken stock (4 cups)
- Cream cheese (4 oz.)
- Crumbled blue cheese (.5 cup + more to serve)

Preparation Technique:
1. Dice the celery and onion.
2. Set the Instant Pot using the sauté mode to warm the oil. Dice/chop and add the celery and onions. Sauté them until they're starting to soften.
3. Measure and shake in the garlic powder and thyme. Sauté the mixture for a couple of minutes.
4. Meanwhile, trim the chicken and remove the skin and bones. Slice it into lengthwise strips.
5. Toss the chicken, hot sauce, and chicken stock into the cooker.

6. Securely close the lid and set the timer for 15 minutes using the high-pressure setting.
7. At that time, natural-release the pressure for ten minutes. Next, quick-release the remainder of the built-up steam.
8. Dice the cream cheese into chunks and crumble the blue cheese.
9. Transfer the chicken to a cutting block to dice/shred it into chunks.
10. Next, mix in both varieties of cheese to the hot soup and wait for it to melt while you're shredding the chicken.
11. Whisk the soup and add the shredded chicken back into the pot.
12. Serve it hot with the blue cheese and hot sauce to your liking

Cauliflower Beef Curry

Servings Provided: 4
Prep & Cook Time: 30 minutes
Macro Counts - Per Serving:
- Calories: 518
- Net Carbohydrates: 3 g
- Fat Content: 34.6 g
- Protein: 44.6 g

Ingredients:
- Cauliflower florets (1 head)
- Ground beef (1.5 lb.)
- Olive oil (2 tbsp.)
- Allspice (.25 tsp.)
- Cumin (.5 tsp.)
- Garlic-ginger paste (1 tbsp.)
- Whole tomatoes (6 oz. can)
- Chili pepper & salt (to your liking)
- Water (.25 cup)

Preparation Technique:
1. Preheat a skillet using the medium-temperature setting to heat the oil.
2. Add the beef to cook for five minutes.
3. Stir in the tomatoes, cauliflower allspice, salt, chili pepper, and cumin. Sauté it for six minutes.
4. Pour in the water and boil for ten minutes.
5. Serve it warm after the liquids have reduced by about half.

Cauliflower & Kielbasa Soup

Servings Provided: 4
Prep & Cook Time: 40 minutes
Macro Counts - Per Serving:
- Calories: 251
- Net Carbohydrates: 5.7 g
- Protein: 10 g
- Fat Content: 19 g

Ingredients:
- Ghee (3 tbsp.)
- Cauliflower (1 head)
- Rutabaga (1)
- Kielbasa sausage (1)
- Chicken broth (2 cups)
- Small onion (1)
- Water (2 cups)
- Black pepper and salt (as desired)

Preparation Technique:
1. Chop the cauliflower, onions, and rutabaga. Slice the sausage.
2. Melt two tablespoons of the ghee in a soup pot. Sauté it for three minutes.
3. Toss in the rutabaga and cauliflower. Sauté it for about five minutes.
4. Pour in the water, broth, pepper, and salt. Boil for about 20 minutes.
5. Melt the butter in a skillet to cook the sausage (5 min.).
6. Puree the soup until it's smooth and serve with the kielbasa.

Chicken Zoodle Soup

Servings Provided: 2
Prep & Cook Time: 15 minutes
Macro Counts - Per Serving:
- Calories: 310
- Net Carbohydrates: 4 g
- Protein: 34 g
- Fat Content: 16 g

Ingredients:
- Chicken breast (1)
- Zucchini (1)
- Avocado oil (2 tbsp.)
- Chicken broth (3 cups)
- Green onion (1)
- Celery stalk (1)
- Cilantro (.25 cup)
- Salt (to your liking)

Preparation Technique:
1. Chop or dice the breast of the chicken. Peel the zucchini.
2. Pour the oil into a saucepan and cook the chicken until done. Pour in the broth and simmer.
3. Chop the celery and green onions and toss into the pan. Simmer for three to four more minutes.
4. Chop the cilantro and prepare the zucchini noodles. Use a potato peeler or spiralizer to make the 'noodles.' Add to the pot.
5. Simmer for a few more minutes and season to taste.

Colby Cauliflower Soup & Pancetta Chips

Servings Provided: 4
Prep & Cook Time: 20 minutes
Macro Counts - Per Serving:
- Calories: 402
- Net Carbohydrates: 6 g
- Protein: 8 g
- Fat Content: 37 g

Ingredients
- Cauliflower florets (2 heads)
- Onion (1)
- Ghee (2 tbsp.)
- Water (2 cups)
- Almond milk (3 cups)
- Shredded Colby cheese (1 cup)
- Pancetta strips (3)

Preparation Technique:
1. Chop the cauliflower and onion. Shred the cheese.
2. Prepare a saucepan and melt the butter. Toss in the onion to sauté for three minutes. Mix in the cauliflower and sauté for three more minutes.
3. Pour in the water, salt, and pepper. Boil and lower the temperature setting to simmer for ten minutes.
4. Puree the cauliflower and stir in the milk and cheese. When it's melted, adjust the seasonings to your liking.
5. Prepare the pancetta until crispy in a skillet. Toss it over the soup and serve.

Creamy Taco Soup

Servings Provided: 4
Prep & Cook Time: 45 minutes
Macro Counts - Per Serving:
- Calories: 347
- Net Carbohydrates: 4 g
- Protein: 21 g
- Fat Content: 27 g

Ingredients:
- Ground chicken/turkey/beef (1 lb.)
- Olive/other cooking oil (1 tbsp.)
- Small onion (1)
- Cloves of garlic (2-3)
- Optional: Green bell pepper (1 small)
- Rotel tomatoes (10 oz. can) or Large tomato (1)
- Cream cheese (8 oz. pkg.) or (Heavy cream (1 cup)
- Taco seasoning (1 pkg.) homemade or (2 tbsp.)
- Salt & pepper (as desired)
- Beef broth (14.5 oz. can/1.5 cups)

Preparation Technique:
1. Add one tablespoon of oil to a large pot. Brown the beef, garlic, and onion using the med-high temperature setting for seven to eight minutes or until the ground beef is browned thoroughly.
2. Dice the garlic, onion, pepper, and tomatoes. Mince the cilantro and set it aside.
3. Mix in the bell pepper, cream cheese, tomatoes, and spices. Stir the mixture for four to five minutes or until the tomatoes are softened and cream cheese is mixed.
4. Dump the beef broth into the soup mixture and lower the heat setting to the medium or low function. Simmer it until the desired thickness is achieved (15-20 min.).
5. Serve it using freshly sliced avocado, jalapenos, sour cream, cilantro, shredded cheese, and a drizzle of lime.

Italian Sausage Soup With Tomatoes & Zucchini Noodles

Servings Provided: 8
Prep & Cook Time: 1 ¾ hours
Macro Counts - Per Serving:
- Calories: 497
- Net Carbohydrates: 4 g
- Protein: 55 g
- Fat Content: 27 g

Ingredients:
- Turkey/pork Italian sausage (19.5 oz. pkg.)
- Olive oil (1 tbsp.)
- Chicken stock (8 cups from a carton/can/homemade)
- Tomato paste (2 tbsp.)
- Petite tomatoes - diced (2 cans/14.5 oz. each)
- Dried basil (1 tbsp.)
- Dried Greek oregano (2 tsp.)
- Optional: Ground fennel (2 tsp.)
- Green and red bell peppers (half of each one)
- Onion (half of one medium)
- Medium zucchini (2 @10-inches long)
- Black pepper & salt (as desired)

Preparation Technique:
1. Chop the onions and peppers.
2. Heat a skillet with a bit of oil and add the sausage to cook until it's browned thoroughly.
3. Combine the sausage, tomato paste, diced tomatoes, chicken stock, and spices into the soup pot. Wait for it to simmer.
4. Dice the bell peppers and onion. Sauté them for a few minutes and toss them into the soup. Simmer them using the low-temperature setting (30-60 min.).
5. Prepare the zucchini into noodles using a veggie peeler or spiralizer. Add them to the soup and simmer on low (20-30 min.).

6. Serve them hot, with a portion of freshly grated parmesan
    as desired.

<u>*Shirataki Soup*</u>

Servings Provided: 2
Prep & Cook Time: 20 minutes
Macro Counts - Per Serving:
- Calories: 130
- Net Carbohydrates: 1.5 g
- Protein: 29.4 g
- Fat Content: 12 g

Ingredients:
- Boneless - skinless chicken thighs (2)
- Chicken stock (3 cups)
- Minced ginger (1 tsp.)
- Cardamom (.25 tsp.)
- Minced garlic (1 clove)
- Mushrooms (.5 cup)
- Optional: Chili sauce (1 tsp.)
- Chopped cilantro (1 pinch)
- Thinly sliced chili pepper (1)

Preparation Technique:
1. Heat the stock on the stovetop using the med-high temperature setting. Toss in the ginger, garlic, mushrooms, and cardamom. Simmer for about ten minutes.
2. Fold in the chicken and cook until done or about five minutes.
3. Prepare two soup bowls and add the sliced chili pepper to each dish. Serve the soup and garnish with some cilantro.
4. Adjust spices as desired.

Chapter 4: Lunchtime & Dinner Side Dish & Bread Specialties

Avocado Tuna Melt Bites

Servings Provided: 12
Prep & Cook Time: 10 minutes
Macro Counts - Per Serving:
- Calories: 185
- Net Carbohydrates: 1 g
- Protein: 5 g
- Fat Content: 17.8 g

Ingredients:
- Mayo (.25 cup)
- Parmesan cheese (.25 cup)
- Drained tuna (10 oz. can)
- Almond flour (.33 cup)
- Onion powder (.25 tsp.)
- Pepper and salt (to your liking)
- Garlic powder (.5 tsp.)
- Cubed avocado (1 medium)
- To Fry: Coconut oil (2 tbsp.)

Preparation Technique:
1. Combine all of the fixings in a bowl - omitting the oil and avocado for now.
2. Fold in the tuna with the cubed avocado. Shape into balls and coat with the flour.
3. Heat the oil using the medium-temperature setting and fry until golden brown to serve.

Cabbage Patties

Servings Provided: 8 patties - 4 servings
Prep & Cook Time: 25 minutes
Macro Counts - Per Serving:
- Net Carbohydrates: 1 g
- Fat Content: 4 g
- Protein: 1 g

Ingredients:
- Cabbage (3 cups) or Egg (1 large)
- Coconut flour (.75 tbsp.)
- Coconut oil, melted (2 tbsp.)
- Optional: Garlic powder & salt

Preparation Technique:
1. Cook and finely chop the cabbage. Toss it with the seasonings and flour into a food processor. Pulse three to four times or until the coconut flour is evenly dispersed.
2. Crack the egg into the mixture and add the oil. Pulse it for another three to four pulses to combine thoroughly. Don't the cabbage too fine.
3. Roll the mixture into eight balls and flatten.
4. Lightly spray a skillet with a cooking oil spray or add additional fat. Add the patties and cook until done.
5. Serve the patties plain or top it off as desired - but count the carbs.

Cool & Spicy Jicama Slaw

Servings Provided: 8
Prep & Cook Time: 8-10 minutes
Macro Counts - Per Serving:
- Net Carbohydrates: 3 g
- Fat Content: 7 g
- Protein: 1 g

Ingredients:
- Julienned jicama (200 g/4 cups)
- Avocado (200 g/1 large)
- Julienned cucumber (200 g/4 cups)
- Radish - sliced thinly (50 g/2 large)
- Grapeseed oil (25 g/2 tbsp.)
- Lime juice (from 1 large lime/25 g/2 tbsp.)
- Optional: Red chili pepper flakes (as desired)

Preparation Technique:
1. Use the widest julienne setting to prepare the jicama and cucumber. Weigh or measure, and combine them in a large mixing container.
2. Use the thinnest setting to slice the radish and toss them with the cucs.
3. Prepare the juice by squeezing the lime and straining any seeds from the juice. Dice the avocado and toss in the juice until coated to help prevent the avocado from premature browning.
4. Toss the avocado with the veggies.
5. If you prefer a creamier slaw, mash the avocado with the juice until smooth, and add the avocado mixture to the jicama. Pour the oil over the mixture, tossing to combine.
6. If using, mix in the chili flakes and wait about ½ hour before serving.

Creamy Green Cabbage

Servings Provided: 4
Prep & Cook Time: 20-25 minutes
Macro Counts - Per Serving:
- Calories: 432
- Net Carbohydrates: 8.2 g
- Protein: 4.2 g
- Fat Content: 42.3 g

Ingredients:
- Butter (2 oz.)
- Shredded green cabbage (1.5 lb.)
- Coconut cream (1.25 cups)
- Finely chopped fresh parsley (8 tbsp.)
- Pepper and salt (as desired)

Preparation Technique:
1. Shred the cabbage and add to a skillet with the butter. Sauté until it's golden brown.
2. Stir in the cream with a sprinkle of salt and pepper. Simmer.
3. Garnish with the parsley and serve while warm.

Creamy Spinach-Rich Ballet

Servings Provided: 4
Prep & Cook Time: 35-40 minutes
Macro Counts - Per Serving:
- Calories: 188
- Net Carbohydrates: 2.9 g
- Protein: 14.6 g
- Fat Content: 12.5 g

Ingredients:
- Fresh baby spinach (1.5 lb.)
- Coconut cream (8 tsp.)
- Sliced cauliflower (14 oz.)
- Melted - unsalted butter (2 tbsp.)
- Black pepper and salt (to your liking)
- Also Needed: 4 ramekins

Preparation Technique:
1. Set the oven temperature at 360° Fahrenheit.
2. Prepare a skillet with the butter. Toss in the spinach to sauté for three minutes.
3. Drain the juices from the spinach and add to the ramekins.
4. Slice the cauliflower and add to the containers with the cream, salt, and pepper.
5. Bake for 25 minutes. Enjoy it warm.

Dried Beef & Cream Cheese Ball

Servings Provided: 10
Prep & Cook Time: varies - 2 hours
Macro Counts - Per Serving:
- Calories: 143
- Net Carbohydrates: 1.1 g
- Protein: 10 g
- Fat Content: 11 g

Ingredients:
- Shredded cheddar cheese (8 oz.)
- Cream cheese (3 oz.)
- Worcestershire sauce (.5 tsp.)
- Black olives (.25 cup)
- Salt: Celery - Garlic & Onion salt (1 pinch each)
- Dried beef (4 oz. jar)

Preparation Technique:
1. Chop the dried beef and set aside.
2. Combine the rest of the fixings. Mix until smooth.
3. Shape into a ball and roll through the beef.
4. Arrange them on a piece of aluminum foil.
5. Refrigerate until ready to serve. Chill overnight or for several hours.

Garlic & Olive Oil Spaghetti Squash

Servings Provided: 2 - main meal or 4 - sides
Prep & Cook Time: 6 minutes
Macro Counts - Per Serving:
- Calories: 181.4
- Net Carbohydrates: 11.6 g
- Protein: 1.7 g
- Fat Content: 14.5 g

Ingredients:
- Spaghetti squash (1)
- Garlic (3-4 cloves)
- Olive oil (2 tbsp.)
- Water (.25 cup)
- Salt and pepper (to your liking)

Preparation Technique:
1. Warm the oven to reach 375° Fahrenheit.
2. Slice the squash in half - lengthwise. Scoop out seeds, saving as much of the inside as possible.
3. Prepare a casserole with a bit of cooking oil spray. Place the squash face-down, and add the water.
4. Bake for ½ hour. Flip the squash and continue cooking for an additional ½ hour - until softened.
5. Mince and sauté the garlic and add the oil in a pan.
6. Grab a serving fork to scrape the squash into the pan. Add the garlic and olive oil.
7. Cook for another three to five minutes with a shake of pepper and salt.

Marinara Zoodles

Servings Provided: 4
Prep & Cook Time: 10-15 minutes
Macro Counts - Per Serving:
- Calories: 179
- Net Carbohydrates: 5.1 g
- Protein: 7 g
- Fat Content: 19 g

Ingredients:
- E-V olive oil (2 tbsp.)
- Garlic cloves (6)
- White onions (.5 cup)
- Tomatoes (14 oz. diced)
- Tomato paste (2 tbsp.)
- Basil leaves (.5 cup roughly-chopped - loosely packed)
- Coarse salt (1.5 tsp.)
- Freshly cracked black pepper (.25 tsp.)
- Cayenne (1 pinch)
- Large zucchini (2 - spiralized)

Preparation Technique:
1. Add the oil to the skillet before placing it on the stovetop (medium-temperature setting).
2. Mince the onion and garlic. Toss them in and sauté the onion for about five minutes before adding in the garlic. Cook for approximately one minute.
3. Mix in the salt, crushed red pepper flakes, pepper, salt, basil, tomato paste, and tomatoes. Combine thoroughly.
4. Simmer the sauce and lower the temperature setting to medium-low. Simmer an additional 15 minutes or until the oil takes on a deep orange color which indicates the sauce is thickened and reduced. Season as desired.
5. Add in the zoodles and let them soften approximately two minutes before serving.

Mushroom & Cauliflower Risotto

Servings Provided: 4
Prep & Cook Time: Under 30 minutes
Macro Counts - Per Serving:
- Calories: 186
- Net Carbohydrates: 4.3 g
- Fat Content: 17.1 g

Ingredients:
- Grated head of cauliflower (1)
- Vegetable stock (1 cup)
- Chopped mushrooms (9 oz.)
- Butter (2 tbsp.)
- Coconut cream (1 cup)
- Pepper and Salt (to taste)

Preparation Technique:
1. Pour the stock in a saucepan. Boil and set aside.
2. Prepare a skillet with butter and saute the mushrooms until golden.
3. Grate and stir in the cauliflower and stock.
4. Simmer and add the cream, cooking until the cauliflower is al dente to serve.

Red Pepper Zoodles

Servings Provided: 4
Prep & Cook Time: 25 minutes
Macro Counts - Per Serving:
- Calories: 198
- Net Carbohydrates: 4.1 g
- Protein: 5 g
- Fat Content: 16.7 g

Ingredients:
- Garlic (1 clove)
- Red bell peppers (1)
- Almond milk (1 cup)
- Olive oil (1 tbsp.)
- Salt (1 tsp.)
- Almond butter (.25 cup)

Preparation Technique:
1. Prepare a baking sheet by lining it with foil.
2. Add the bell peppers to the baking sheet before placing them on the top level of your broiler and letting them cook until blackened. Remove and cool.
3. Once they have cooled you can remove the skins, stems, seeds, and ribs.
4. Add the prepared mixture, along with the remaining sauce ingredients, and blend thoroughly. Season as desired.
5. Serve with zoodles as well as a variety of potential toppings including things like truffle oil, goat cheese, or parsley.

Stuffed Mushrooms

Servings Provided: 4
Prep & Cook Time: 30 minutes
Macro Counts - Per Serving:
- Calories: 124
- Net Carbohydrates: 2.6 g
- Protein: 5 g
- Fat Content: 22.4 g

Ingredients:
- Portobello mushrooms (4)
- Blue cheese (1 cup)
- Olive oil (2 tbsp.)
- Fresh thyme (1 pinch)
- Salt (as desired)

Preparation Technique:
1. Set the oven temperature at 350° Fahrenheit.
2. Cut the stems from the mushrooms and chop them to bits.
3. Mix with the thyme, salt, and crumbled blue cheese and stuff the mushrooms.
4. Spritz with some of the oil.
5. Bake for 15-20 minutes.
6. Serve it piping hot.

Zucchini Noodle Gratin

Servings Provided: 8
Prep & Cook Time: 1 ¾ hours
Macro Counts - Per Serving:
- Calories: 200
- Net Carbohydrates: 3 g
- Protein: 6 g
- Fat Content: 18 g

Ingredients:
- Loosely packed zucchini noodles (8 cups/800 g)
- Heavy cream (1 cup/238 g)
- Shredded Gruyere cheese (4 oz./113 g)
- Butter (3 tbsp./42 g)
  Optional Seasonings:
- Black pepper
- Salt
- Garlic powder
- Fresh herbs
- Also Needed: 9-inch baking dish

Preparation Technique:
1. Make the zucchini noodles and place them in a mesh colander. Grab and garnish using the salt and toss to coat evenly. Leave them in the sink for about two hours to release moisture. Gently dry and squeeze the excess moisture from the noodles with a paper towel.
2. Warm the oven to reach 350° Fahrenheit. Lightly grease the baking dish with butter and add the noodles in an even layer.
3. Use a saucepan to combine the butter, heavy cream, and cheese. Warm the mixture using the medium-temperature setting until melted and the sauce is smooth. Transfer the pan to a cool burner and add optional seasonings.
4. Pour the cream mixture over the noodles and bake for about one hour or until nicely browned.

5. Cool the gratin for about 15 minutes and slice into eight
   portions to serve.

Flatbread Specialties

Buttery Low-Carb Flatbread

Servings Provided: 4
Prep & Cook Time: 7 minutes
Macro Counts - Per Serving:
- Calories: 232
- Net Carbohydrates: 4 g
- Protein: 9 g
- Fat Content: 19 g

Ingredients:
- Almond flour (1 cup)
- Xanthan gum (2 tsp.)
- Coconut flour (2 tsp.)
- Baking powder (.5 tsp.)
- Falk salt (.5 tsp.)
- Eggs (1 whole + 1 white)
- Water (1 tbsp.)
- Oil for frying (1 tbsp.)
- Melted butter - for slathering (1 tbsp./to your liking)

Preparation Technique:
1. Whisk the dry fixings (baking powder, salt, flours, and xanthan gum) until fully blended.
2. Whisk and add the egg and egg white. Gently beat into the flour. The dough will begin to form.
3. Pour the water and begin to work the dough for the flour and xanthan gum to absorb the moisture.
4. Portion the dough into four equal parts and press each section out with cling wrap.
5. Add the oil into a large skillet using the medium temperature setting on the stovetop. Fry each flatbread for about one minute per side.
6. Brush with butter. Garnish with salt and chopped parsley.

Indian Cuisine Naan Bread

Servings Provided: 6
Prep & Cook Time: 17-20 minutes
Macro Counts - Per Serving:
- Calories: 91
- Net Carbohydrates: 3.6 g
- Protein: 3.5 g
- Fat Content: 6.4 g

Ingredients:
Dry Ingredients
- Coconut flour (.75 cup)
- Psyllium husk powder (2 tbsp.)
- Xanthan gum (1 tsp.)
- Salt (1 generous pinch)
- Baking powder (1 tsp.)
- Sesame seeds (1 tbsp.)
Wet Ingredients:
- Hot water (1 cup)
- Full-fat natural yogurt (.25 cup)
- Coconut oil/olive oil melted (2 tbsp.)
Topping Ingredients:
- Coconut oil/butter/olive oil - heated (2 tbsp.)
- Chopped parsley or coriander/cilantro (handful)
- Salt (1 generous pinch)

Preparation Technique:
1. Warm the oven to reach 356° Fahrenheit.
2. Combine the dry fixings in a mixing container - removing all of the lumps.
3. Mix in the wet components and work into a dough ball.
4. Wait for a few minutes and divide the dough into six pieces. Roll them out between two sheets of parchment paper into long flatbreads. Place on an upturned baking sheet and remove the top parchment. Garnish using sesame seeds.

5. Bake 12-15 minutes until they are the way you like them.
    Garnish as desired.

Rosemary - Oregano & Thyme Flatbread

Servings Provided: 1
Prep & Cook Time: 30 minutes
Macro Counts - Per Serving:
- Calories: 703
- Net Carbohydrates: 16 g
- Protein: 42 g
- Fat Content: 52 g

Ingredients:
- Shredded mozzarella cheese (1 cup)
- Cream cheese (1 tbsp.)
- Large egg (1)
- Almond flour (.25 cup)
- Fresh rosemary (1 tsp.)
- Cloves of garlic (2)
- Dried oregano (.5 tsp.)
- Dried thyme (.5 tsp.)
- Black pepper and salt (to your liking)

Preparation Technique:
1. Mince the rosemary and garlic.
2. Heat the oven to 350° Fahrenheit. Cover a baking tin with a layer of parchment baking paper or a spritz of cooking oil spray.
3. Combine both types of cheese. Microwave at 30-second intervals. Stir between the intervals until the cheese is melted and the consistency is smooth (approximately one minute).
4. Cool for a few minutes. Add the egg, salt, garlic, oregano, rosemary, almond flour, thyme, and pepper, and stir until fully mixed.
5. Scoop onto the baking sheet. Press into an even layer about 0.5-inch thick.
6. Bake for 10 to 15 minutes. Serve.

Are you enjoying this book? If so, I'd love to hear your feedback: leave an honest review on Amazon, it means a lot to me and motivates me to do better and better! Thank you!

Chapter 5: Seafood Specialties

Crab Cakes

Servings Provided: 3
Prep & Cook Time: 12 minutes
Macro Counts - Per Serving:
- Net Carbohydrates: 4 g
- Protein: 25 g
- Fat Content: 43 g

Ingredients:
- Crabmeat (.33 cup/87 g from blue crabs)
- Almond flour -ex. - Bob's Red Mill (.25 cup/25 g)
- Mayo - ex. - Trader Joe's Organic (2 heaping tbsp./ 35 g)
- Raw large egg (1/25 g)
- Raw green onion - tops only - thinly sliced (1 tbsp.)
- Ground - dried mustard (.25 tsp.)
- Salt/pepper/garlic powder (as desired)

Preparation Technique:
1. Thoroughly clean the crab meat and mix it with the rest of the fixings.
2. Lightly grease a skillet with a spritz of cooking oil spray and warm it using the med-high temperature setting.
3. Portion the mixture into three equal patties and arrange them in the pan. Cook the first side for about two to three minutes or until browned and sides are beginning to set.
4. Turn the crab cakes over and continue cooking for an additional two to three minutes or until it's thoroughly cooked.
5. Serve with greens and mayonnaise-based dressing as desired, but count those carbs.

Crunchy Fish and Chaffle Bites

Servings Provided: 4
Prep & Cook Time: 15-20 minutes
Macro Counts - Per Serving:
- Calories: 321
- Net Carbohydrates: 1.3 g
- Protein: 28.7 g
- Fat Content: 21.4 g

Ingredients:
- Cod fillets (1 lb./4 slices)
- Garlic powder (1 tsp.)
- Sea salt (1 tsp.)
- Whisked egg (1)
- Almond flour (1 cup)
- Avocado oil (2 tsp.)
    The Chaffles:
- Cheddar cheese (.5 cup)
- Eggs (2)
- Italian seasoning (.5 tsp.)
- Almond flour (2 tbsp.)

Preparation Technique:
1. Whisk the chaffle fixings and warm the mini waffle maker.
2. Pour the batter into the heated waffle iron.
3. Whisk the garlic powder, pepper, and salt. Add the cod to the mixture and wait for about ten minutes.
4. At that point, dip them into the almond flour.
5. Warm the oil in a skillet and fry the fish for two to three minutes. Serve the delicious fish with the chaffles.

Mediterranean Grilled Ahi Tuna

Servings Provided: 4
Prep & Cook Time: 25 minutes
Macro Counts - Per Serving:
- Calories: 229.2
- Net Carbohydrates: 0.4 g
- Protein: 42.5 g
- Fat Content: 5.3 g

Ingredients:
- Ahi Tuna Steaks (1-inch thick - 4 @ 5 oz. each - Uncooked fresh or frozen-thawed)
- E-V olive oil (1 tbsp.)
- Black pepper (.25 tsp.)
- Kosher salt (.5 tsp.)
- Lemon juice (1 lemon wedge/.5 tsp.)
- Finely chopped oregano (.5 tsp.) _or_ dried (.25 tsp.)
- Red pepper flakes (.25 tsp.) _or_ crushed/dried (a dash)
- Fresh basil (1 tsp.) _or_ dried (.25 tsp.)
- Garlic (1 clove)

Preparation Technique:
1. Preheat an outside grill using the med-high temperature setting, or start the charcoal grill for about 30 minutes.
2. Remove excess moisture from the steaks using paper towels and place them into a shallow dish.
3. Finely mince the garlic. Whisk the spices with oil and lemon juice. Wait for at least five minutes to blend the flavors.
4. Brush the mixture on both sides of the steaks and wait another five minutes.
5. Grill the tuna steaks for two to five minutes on each side. Rare is most preferred with a slightly pink center.

Parmesan Crusted Tilapia

Servings Provided: 4
Prep & Cook Time: 20 minutes
Macro Counts - Per Serving:
- Calories: 202.9
- Net Carbohydrates: 0.2 g
- Protein: 23.7 g
- Fat Content: 11.5 g

Ingredients:
- Tilapia filets (4 @ 4 oz. each)
- Parmesan (.25 cup)
- Unchilled butter (3 tbsp.)
- Lemon juice (2 tsp.)
- Salt & black pepper (to your liking)

Preparation Technique:
1. Sprinkle the fish using pepper and salt.
2. Combine the cheese with the butter, salt, pepper, and lemon juice.
3. Arrange the tilapia on a baking tray sprayed with a spritz of cooking oil spray. Cover the fish with the cheese mixture and broil until it is golden brown.
4. Serve hot over a batch of Spanish rice - but add the carbs.

Parmesan Shrimp

Servings Provided: 2
Prep & Cook Time: 20 minutes
Macro Counts - Per Serving:
- Calories: 137.6
- Net Carbohydrates: 4.5 g
- Protein: 10.2 g
- Fat Content: 8.6 g

Ingredients:
- Shrimp (14 medium/26-30 per lb. count)
- Olive oil (1 tbsp.)
- Garlic (half of 1 clove)
- Light salt (2 dashes)
- Creole seasoning (.25 tsp.)
- Fresh ground pepper (2 dashes)
- Panko breadcrumbs (.125 cup or ⅛ cup)
- Shredded parmesan cheese (1 tbsp.)
- Optional: Lemon wedges
- Butter-flavored/keto-friendly cooking spray (as needed)
- Also Needed: 8x8 baking pan

Preparation Technique:
1. You can use either - fresh and thawed pre-peeled shrimp. Mince the garlic.
2. Peel and devein the shrimp and toss them into a zipper-type bag with the garlic, olive oil, salt, pepper, and creole seasoning. Gently flip the bag in all directions until the shrimp is well coated.
3. Place the bag in the fridge for 30 minutes to one hour.
4. Warm the oven at 475° Fahrenheit.
5. Toss the breadcrumbs and parmesan into the baggie and gently turn to coat.
6. Arrange the shrimp in a single layer into the ungreased pan so they're not touching. Spritz the baking tray using the cooking spray.

7. Broil for approximately ten minutes until done. Serve promptly.
8. Garnish with lemon wedges as desired (add the carbs).
9. Note: The prep time doesn't include ½ hour to marinate or to peel the shrimp.

Salmon Cakes

Servings Provided: 4
Prep & Cook Time: 30 minutes
Macro Counts - Per Serving:
- Calories: 195
- Net Carbohydrates: 3.6 g
- Protein: 23.2 g
- Fat Content: 10.1 g

Ingredients:
- Wild Alaskan Pink Salmon - ex. - Bumble Bee (14.75 oz. can)
- Raw onion (1 cup + more if desired)
- Garlic powder (1 tsp.)
- Large egg (1)
- Black pepper (1 tsp.)
- Salt (as desired)
- Butter or other fat - to fry

Preparation Technique:
1. Mix all of the fixings to form four patties.
2. Fry patties as you would a hamburger in a bit of butter for flavoring.
3. Serve with your favorite sides or in a sandwich.

Shrimp Scampi

Servings Provided: 4
Prep & Cook Time: 15 minutes
Macro Counts - Per Serving:
- Calories: 143.2
- Net Carbohydrates: 1.9 g
- Fat Content: 6.1 g
- Protein: 19 g

Ingredients:
- Canola oil (1 tbsp.)
- Uncooked shrimp (.75 lb.)
- Green onion (1 medium)
- Garlic powder (.25 tsp.)
- Basil (.5 tsp.)
- Parsley (.75 tsp.)
- Lemon juice (1 tbsp.)
- Parmesan cheese (3 tbsp.)
- Also Needed: 10-inch skillet

Preparation Technique:
1. Prepare the oil in the skillet using the med-high temperature setting.
2. Dice the onion. Peel, devein, and toss the shrimp with the rest of the fixings.
3. Cook for three to seven minutes.
4. When ready, dust with the parmesan cheese to serve.
5. Note: If the shrimp is cooked into an 'o' shape, it is overcooked; stick with the shape of a 'c' for a guideline.

Shrimp Scampi For Garlic Lovers

Servings Provided: 6
Prep & Cook Time: 15 minutes
Macro Counts - Per Serving:
- Calories: 120.5
- Net Carbohydrates: 1.2 g
- Fat Content: 5.4 g
- Protein: 16 g

Ingredients:
- Frozen - defrosted/fresh shrimp (1 lb.)
- Garlic (5 cloves + more if desired)
- Olive oil (1/8 cup)
- Parsley (2 tbsp. + more for garnish)
- To Serve: Lemon juice (1 lemon + lemon wedges for serving
- Black pepper & salt (1 tsp. each)

Preparation Technique:
1. Warm the oil using the low-temperature setting. Mince and add the garlic and sauté it until golden. Adjust the temperature setting to med-high.
2. Toss in the shrimp, salt, pepper, and parsley. Flip the shrimp over once the bottom side is pink.
3. Cook on the second side until pink on the outside and opaque throughout (10 min.).
4. Mix in lemon juice and simmer for ½ minute more. Remove the pan from the burner and serve promptly with a portion of parsley and lemon wedges.

Chapter 6: Poultry Specialties

Balsamic Grilled Chicken Breast

Servings Provided: 8
Prep & Cook Time: 50 minutes
Macro Counts - Per Serving:
- Calories: 210
- Net Carbohydrates: 2.6 g
- Protein: 26 g
- Fat Content: 9.8 g

Ingredients:
- Chicken breast - fresh or frozen (8 @ 4 oz. each)
- Water (1 cup)
- Olive oil (.5 cup)
- Balsamic vinegar (2 tbsp.)
- Dried onion flakes (4 tsp.)
- Italian seasoning (3 tsp.)
- Ground mustard (3 tsp.)
- Thyme (2 tsp.)
- Black pepper & salt (2 tsp. each)

Preparation Technique:
1. Whisk the olive oil with the balsamic vinegar, thyme, Italian seasoning, pepper, salt, and onion flakes. Pour it into a one-gallon resealable plastic zipper-type bag.
2. Trim the chicken from all fat and bones. Toss it into the bag.
3. Marinate the chicken for at least 30 minutes.
4. Warm the grill. Add the chicken and sear both sides. Grill it until the meat is white throughout or has an internal temp of 180° Fahrenheit.

Chicken Nuggets

Servings Provided: 24 nuggets @ 6 servings
Prep & Cook Time: 45 minutes
Macro Counts - Per Serving:
- Calories: 2124
- Net Carbohydrates: 11 g
- Protein: 65 g
- Fat Content: 203 g

Ingredients:
- Chicken breast (2 cups)
- Coconut flour (.25 cup)
- Sir Kensington's Avocado oil (.5 cup)
- Mayonnaise (.5 cup)
- Fresh egg (1 large/50g)
- Salt/pepper (as desired)

Preparation Technique:
1. Finely shred and combine the chicken with the coconut flour and seasonings. Use a fork to combine the fixings, evenly distributing and coating the chicken with the dry components.
2. Fold in the avocado oil, mayo, and egg. Stir to combine until it's similar to a pancake mix.
3. Wait a few minutes to warm a skillet using the medium-high temperature setting.
4. Drop spoonfuls of the batter and fry as you would pancakes, flipping at least once.
5. Once the nuggets have thoroughly cooked, leave them in the pan to cool and absorb the oil, or scrape the pan and drizzle the oil over the nuggets.
6. Serve them promptly. You can freeze the nuggets in a single layer and add to a freezer container or plastic bag.
7. To reheat, place the frozen nuggets in a pan and heat until thawed using the med-low temperature setting.
8. Alternatively, warm the oven to reach 450° Fahrenheit. Bake the nuggets in cupcake tins for about 15 to 20

minutes. Cool in the molds to reabsorb fat that has cooked out.

Creamy Chicken Broccoli

Servings Provided: 1
Prep & Cook Time: 26 minutes
Macro Counts - Per Serving:
- Calories: 500
- Net Carbohydrates: 5 g
- Protein: 18 g
- Fat Content: 46 g

Ingredients:
- 36% heavy cream (40 grams or 1/3 cup)
- Broccoli - raw (80 grams/approx. 1 cup)
- Lemon juice 100% - bottled or fresh (1 tsp.)
- Large chicken breast - raw, skinless, cut into small pieces (70 grams/about 1/3 of a breast)
- Butter (2 tbsp.)
- Olive oil (1.5 tbsp.)
- For Thinning: Chicken broth - 100% Natural - Swanson
- Optional: Tabasco sauce (to your liking)

Preparation Technique:
1. Melt the butter with the olive oil in a small skillet using the med-high temperature setting.
2. Carefully trim the chicken into bite-sized chunks and add it to the pan. Sauté for three minutes, turning the chicken to brown.
3. Reduce the temperature to medium. Mix in the lemon juice, a dash of black pepper, Tabasco sauce, and salt - stirring until coated.
4. Chop the broccoli into bite-sized pieces. Stir in cream and broccoli. Simmer for two to three more minutes while stirring.
5. Stir in chicken broth and cover the pan. Turn off the burner and let it rest about ten minutes to finish cooking the broccoli and chicken.

Fiesta Lime Chicken

Servings Provided: 8 @ ½ breast each serving
Prep & Cook Time: 17 minutes
Macro Counts - Per Serving:
- Calories: 208.9
- Net Carbohydrates: 5.6 g
- Protein: 31.4 g
- Fat Content: 6.2 g

Ingredients:
- Chicken breast (4 - cut in half)
- Garlic (3 cloves)
- Juice (1.5 limes)
- Salsa (1 cup)
- Reduced-fat ranch dressing (.25 cup)
- Cheddar cheese - reduced-fat (1 cup - shredded)

Preparation Technique:
1. Trim the chicken, making sure all fat and bones are removed.
2. Lightly spritz a skillet with cooking oil spray and heat using the medium-temperature setting.
3. Sauté the chicken for three minutes on each side. Mince and toss in the garlic.
4. Whisk the salsa, lime juice, and ranch dressing in a mixing container. Spread it over the top of the chicken. Simmer for an additional five minutes.
5. Garnish it with the cheese, cover, and cook until the chicken is no longer pink (4-5 min.).

Parmesan Chicken

Servings Provided: 1
Prep & Cook Time: 35 minutes
Macro Counts - Per Serving:
- Calories: 190.6
- Net Carbohydrates: 0.4 g
- Fat Content: 7 g
- Protein: 29.2 g

Ingredients:
- Chicken breast (1)
- Dijon mustard (1 tsp.)
- Grated parmesan cheese (2 tbsp.)
- Cooking oil spray

Preparation Technique:
1. Trim the fat and bones from the chicken breasts.
2. Brush the chicken with the dijon mustard evenly on both sides.
3. Pat cheese onto the chicken to create a crust.
4. Arrange it on a baking tray. Lightly spritz it using the cooking spray to help make it golden brown and crusty.
5. Bake at 375° Fahrenheit for 20 to 30 minutes and serve as desired.

Quick & Easy Creamy Mushroom Chicken

Servings Provided: 6
Prep & Cook Time: 45 minutes
Macro Counts - Per Serving:
- Calories: 223.8
- Net Carbohydrates: 5.8 g
- Protein: 29.7 g
- Fat Content: 7.9 g

Ingredients:
- Boneless & skinless chicken breast or tenderloins - diced (1.5 lb.)
- Low-sodium chicken broth (2 cups)
- Cream of Mushroom *or* Cream of Chicken Soup - ex. - Campbell's Healthy Request (2 small cans)
- Neufchatel low-fat cream cheese (3 oz.)
- Freshly snipped chives (4 tbsp.) or (can use dry also)
- Mushrooms - drained (1 cup - canned)

Preparation Technique:
1. Drain the mushrooms and set aside.
2. Prepare a large - high sided skillet with the broth and diced chicken breast.
3. Set the temperature to high. Once boiling, adjust the temperature setting to med-high. Continue cooking chicken, occasionally stirring, for about ½ hour until it's no longer pink inside.
4. Mix in the cream of mushroom soup, mushrooms, and Neufchatel cream cheese. Mix well until cream cheese is melted, all of the fixings are incorporated, and the mixture is hot (5-10 min.)
5. Serve as is or with a serving of noodles or rice.

Chapter 7: Pork - Lamb & Beef Specialties

Pork Options

Asian-Inspired Pork Chops

Servings Provided: 3
Prep & Cook Time: 20 minutes
Macro Counts - Per Serving:
- Calories: 106.1
- Net Carbohydrates: 2.7 g
- Protein: 11.5 g
- Fat Content: 5.5 g

Ingredients:
- Pork chops (3 thinly-sliced center cut)
- Bragg Liquid Aminos/Sub. for soy sauce/or another favorite keto-friendly (2 tbsp.)
- Garlic powder (.5 tsp.)
- Salt (1 pinch)
- Black pepper (.5 tsp.)
- Ginger (.5 tsp.)
- Minced garlic (2 tsp.)
- Diced onions (1 tbsp.)

Preparation Technique:
1. Mince the garlic and dice the onions. Toss everything into a zipper-type plastic bag. Shake the fixings.
2. Put the pork chops in a bag. Marinate two to 24 hours in the fridge, turning the bag from time to time.
3. Discard the marinade and drain the meat.
4. Grill them for 12-15 minutes using the medium temperature setting or until the desired doneness.

Crockpot Pork Chops

Servings Provided: 10
Prep & Cook Time: 7-9 hours
Macro Counts - Per Serving:
- Calories: 239.7
- Net Carbohydrates: 7.7 g
- Protein: 21.8 g
- Fat Content: 12.1 g

Ingredients:
- Pork chops (Family pack - about 10)
- Low-sodium/low-fat cream/mushroom/chicken celery, etc. (1 can)
- Ketchup (.5 cup)

Preparation Technique:
1. Arrange the chops in the cooker. Add the ketchup and soup of choice.
2. Stir and close the lid. Place the timer on for seven to nine hours on the low setting.

Hot Tex-Mex Pork Casserole

Servings Provided: 4
Prep & Cook Time: 35 minutes
Macro Counts - Per Serving:
- Calories: 431
- Net Carbohydrates: 7.8 g
- Protein: 43 g
- Fat Content: 24 g

Ingredients:
- Butter (2 tbsp.)
- Ground pork (1.5 lb.)
- Tex-Mex seasoning (3 tbsp.)
- Jalapenos (2 tbsp.)
- Monterey jack shredded cheese (.5 cup)
- Crushed tomatoes (.5 cup)
- _Serving & Garnish:_
- Scallion (1)
- Sour cream (1 cup)

Preparation Technique:
1. Warm the oven to reach 330° Fahrenheit.
2. Lightly spritz a baking tray using a cooking oil spray.
3. Add the butter to a skillet with the pork, and cook it for about eight minutes or until browned. Add the jalapenos, Tex-Mex, pepper, salt, and tomatoes. Simmer it for about five minutes.
4. Dump the fixings into the prepared dish and drizzle it with the cheese.
5. Set the timer for 20 minutes until it's golden brown.
6. Garnish as desired.

Maple Country-Style Pork Ribs - Slow-Cooked

Servings Provided: 4
Prep & Cook Time: 7-9 hours
Macro Counts - Per Serving:
- Calories: 188.4
- Net Carbohydrates: 2 g
- Protein: 22.3 g
- Fat Content: 9.4 g

Ingredients:
- Ground allspice (.25 tsp.)
- Ground cinnamon (.25 tsp.)
- Country-style pork ribs (2 lb. before cooked - will yield 16 oz. meat)
- Onion (.25 cup)
- Garlic powder (.5 tsp.)
- Maple-flavored syrup- no sugar (1 tbsp.)
- Black pepper (1 dash)
- Ground ginger (.25 tsp.)
- Low-sodium soy sauce (1 tbsp.)

Preparation Technique:
1. Dice the onion and measure the rest of the components. Toss all of the fixings except for the ribs into a mixing container.
2. Pour the sauce over the ribs.
3. Pop it into a crockpot to cook with the lid 'on' using the low setting for seven to nine hours.

Lamb Options

Lamb & Asparagus with Tangy Sauce

Servings Provided: 1
Prep & Cook Time: 30 minutes
Macro Counts - Per Serving:
- Calories: 500
- Net Carbohydrates: 3.7 g
- Protein: 15 g
- Fat Content: 47 g

Ingredients:
- Olive oil (1 tbsp.)
- Orange juice - unsweetened (1 tsp.)
- Lime juice - unsweetened (1 tsp.)
- Garlic (1 minced clove)
- Curry powder (1 tsp.)
- Raw lamb shoulder (80 grams)
- Asparagus - raw (.5 cup)

Preparation Technique:
1. Mince and add the garlic with the curry powder, orange juice, and lime juice to make the marinade.
2. Cut a one-inch slice of lamb shoulder to the appropriate servings size for one serving and place it in a small bowl with the marinade sauce. Pop it into the fridge for two to four hours.
3. Use an eight-inch square piece of foil and place it on a shallow oven-proof dish. Arrange the lamb on the foil and surround it with the asparagus spears. Broil it for six to eight minutes -rotating it once. Remove the asparagus as they are browned.
4. Meanwhile, warm the oil in a small saucepan. Pour in the marinade and simmer until the mixture has thickened. Transfer the cooked asparagus and lamb to the pan and turn off the heat. Wait a few minutes and serve.

Kofta Kebab

Servings Provided: 16 kebabs
Prep & Cook Time: 40 minutes
Macro Counts - Per Serving:
- Calories: 145
- Net Carbohydrates: 1 g
- Fat Content: 11 g
- Protein: 10 g

Ingredients:
- Ground lamb (1 lb.)
- 85% ground beef (1 lb.)
- Yellow onion (.5 cup)
- Fresh parsley (1 cup)
- Garlic (2 cloves)
- Black pepper & salt
  Spices Used - 1 tsp. Each:
- Ground nutmeg (1 tsp.)
- Sumac
- Ground green cardamom
- Ground allspice
- Also Needed: 16 wooden skewers

Preparation Technique:
1. Soak the skewers in water for at least one hour before it's time to grill.
2. Chop the onion, garlic, and parsley.
3. Toss all of the fixings into a large mixing container. Fold the spices into the meat mixture using your hands until it's thoroughly combined.
4. Portion the meat into ¼-cup portions and press them onto the skewer in a log shape.
5. Grill the kebabs until the internal temperature reaches 160° Fahrenheit, and it's nicely browned. Remove the kebabs from the grill, cover with foil, and wait for at least five minutes before serving.

6. Serve with grilled vegetables and our Tzatziki sauce for a delicious meal.

Roasted Leg of Lamb

Servings Provided: 6
Prep & Cook Time: 2 hours - varies
Macro Counts - Per Serving:
- Net Carbohydrates: 1 g
- Calories: 223
- Fat Content: 14 g
- Protein: 22 g

Ingredients:
- Reduced-sodium beef broth (.5 cup)
- Leg of lamb (2 lb.)
- Chopped garlic cloves (6)
- Fresh rosemary leaves (1 tbsp.)
- Black pepper (1 tsp.)

Preparation Technique:
1. Grease a baking pan and set the oven temperature to 400° Fahrenheit.
2. Arrange the lamb in the pan and add the broth and seasonings.
3. Roast 30 minutes and lower the heat to 350° Fahrenheit. Continue cooking for about one hour or until done.
4. Let the lamb stand about 20 minutes before slicing to serve.
5. Enjoy with some roasted brussels sprouts and extra rosemary for a tasty change of pace.

Beef Options

Bacon Burger & Cabbage Stir Fry

Servings Provided: 10
Prep & Cook Time: 20 minutes
Macro Counts - Per Serving:
- Calories: 357
- Net Carbohydrates: 4.5 g
- Protein: 32 g
- Fat Content: 22 g

Ingredients:
- Ground beef (1 lb.)
- Bacon (1 lb.)
- Small onion (1)
- Minced cloves of garlic (3)
- Cabbage (1 lb. - 1 small head)
- Black pepper (.25 tsp.)
- Sea salt (.5 tsp.)

Preparation Technique:
1. Dice the bacon and onion.
2. Combine the beef and bacon in a wok or large skillet. Prepare until done and store in a bowl to keep warm.
3. Mince the onion and garlic. Toss both into the hot grease.
4. Slice and toss in the cabbage and stir-fry until wilted.
5. Blend in the meat and combine. Sprinkle with the pepper and salt as desired.

BBQ Flank Steak

Servings Provided: 8
Prep & Cook Time: 8 hours
Macro Counts - Per Serving:
- Calories: 342
- Net Carbohydrates: 1 g
- Protein: 35 g
- Fat Content: 21 g

Ingredients:
- Flank steak (3 lb.)
- Paprika (1 tsp.)
- Granulated garlic (1 tsp.)
- Cayenne pepper (1 tsp.)
- Granulated onion (1 tsp.)
- White pepper (1 tsp.)
- Salt (1 tsp.)
- Black pepper (1 tsp.)
- Coconut aminos (1 tbsp.)
- Water (.25 cup)
- Melted butter (2 tbsp.)
- Also Needed: Slow cooker

Preparation Technique:
1. Combine the seasonings, aminos, and melted butter. Rub into the steak.
2. Add the water to the cooker and the steak fixings.
3. Cook for 8 hours (flip ½ through the cooking cycle).
4. Serve with some creamy spinach.

Cabbage Rolls - Slow Cooked

Servings Provided: 3 rolls each - 5 servings
Prep & Cook Time: 6 hours 10 minutes
Macro Counts - Per Serving:
- Calories: 481
- Net Carbohydrates: 4 g
- Protein: 35 g
- Fat Content: 25 g

Ingredients:
- Corned beef (3.5 lb.)
- Large savoy cabbage leaves (15)
- White wine (.25 cup)
- Coffee (.25 cup)
- Large lemon (1)
- Medium sliced onion (1)
- Rendered bacon fat (1 tbsp.)
- Erythritol (1 tbsp.)
- Yellow mustard (1 tbsp.)
- Large bay leaf (1)
- Kosher salt (2 tsp.)
- Cloves (.25 tsp.)
- Allspice (.25 tsp.)
- Red pepper flakes (.5 tsp.)
- Whole peppercorns (1 tsp.)
- Mustard seeds (1 tsp.)
- Worcestershire sauce (2 tsp.)

Preparation Technique:
1. Pour the liquids, corned beef, and spices into the cooker. Set the timer for six hours using the low setting.
2. Prepare a pot of boiling water. When the timer on the slow cooker buzzes, add the leaves along with the sliced onion to the water for two to three minutes. Transfer the leaves to a cold-water bath. Blanch them for three to four minutes. Continue boiling the onion.
3. Use a paper towel to dry the leaves. Add the onions and

beef.

4. Roll up the cabbage leaves. Drizzle with freshly squeezed lemon juice. Serve any time.

Creamy Burrito Bake

Servings Provided: 8
Prep & Cook Time: 40 minutes
Macro Counts - Per Serving:
- Calories: 383
- Net Carbohydrates: 9.9 g
- Protein: 23 g
- Fat Content: 27.6 g
-

Ingredients:
- Lean ground beef (1 lb.)
- Old El Paso Taco Seasoning (1 package)
- Monterey jack cheese (8 oz - grated)
- Cream of mushroom soup (1 small)
- Sour cream (.5 cup)
- Taco Bell Taco Sauce - mild (4oz./half a jar)
- Low-carb tortilla - ex. - La Tortilla Factory (8)
- Also Needed: 9 x 12 baking pan

Preparation Technique:
1. Brown the beef and mix in the taco seasoning. Prepare it according to package directions.
2. Whisk the can of soup with the sour cream and taco sauce.
3. Spritz the pan using a cooking oil spray and spoon one-third of the soup mixture into the pan. Portion the meat mixture into the tortillas and sprinkle cheese in the shell before folding and placing it in the pan.
4. Reserve about ½ to ¾ of a cup of cheese.
5. Spread the remainder of the soup mixture over the shells and top with the rest of the cheese.
6. Bake at 350° Fahrenheit until bubbly, and the cheese is melted (20-25 min.).

Mississippi Pot Roast

Servings Provided: 8
Prep & Cook Time: 8-10 hours
Macro Counts - Per Serving:
- Calories: 435
- Net Carbohydrates: 3 g
- Protein: 33 g
- Fat Content: 32 g

Ingredients:
- Deli-sliced peperoncini (16 oz. jar)
- Beef chuck roast (3.8 lb.)
- Salt (.5 tsp.)
- Dried dill (1 tbsp.)
- Garlic powder (1 tbsp.)
- Dried chives (1 tbsp.)
- Onion powder (1 tbsp.)
- Dried parsley (1 tbsp.)
- Black pepper (.25 tsp.)
- Better than Bouillon (2 tbsp.)
- Also Needed: Slow Cooker

Preparation Technique:
1. Drain the pepperoncini – reserving the brine.
2. Set the cooker on the high-temperature setting. Add the roast and pepperoncini. Pour one cup of the brine into the cooker and trash the rest.
3. Stir in the bouillon paste and spices. Lastly, add the stick of butter.
4. Prepare using the high setting for eight to ten hours. You don't need to stir.
5. When the roast is done and falling away from the bone, shred it with a fork and serve.

Nacho Skillet Steak

Servings Provided: 5
Prep & Cook Time: 55-60 minutes
Macro Counts - Per Serving:
- Calories: 385
- Net Carbohydrates: 6 g
- Protein: 19 g
- Fat Content: 31 g

Ingredients:
- Cauliflower (1.5 lb.)
- Turmeric (.5 tsp.)
- Chili powder (1 tsp.)
- Butter (1 tbsp.)
- Beef round tip steak (8 oz.)
- Melted refined coconut oil (.33 cup)
- Shredded Monterey Jack & Cheddar cheese (1 oz. each)
  Optional Garnishes:
- Sour cream (.33 cup)
- Canned - jalapeno slices (1 oz.)
- Avocado (approx. 5 oz.)

Preparation Technique:
1. Warm the oven temperature to 400° Fahrenheit.
2. Prepare the cauliflower into chip-like shapes.
3. Combine the turmeric, chili powder, and coconut oil in a mixing dish.
4. Toss in the cauliflower and add it to a baking tin. Set the baking timer for 20 to 25 minutes.
5. Over med-high heat in a cast-iron skillet, add the butter. Cook until both sides of the meat are done, flipping just once. Let it rest for 5-10 minutes. Thinly slice and sprinkle with some pepper and salt.
6. When done, transfer the florets to the skillet and add the steak strips. Top it off with the cheese and bake for 5-10 more minutes.
7. Serve with your favorite garnish.

8. Count the carbs for the added garnishes.

Skillet Cabbage Tacos

Servings Provided: 4
Prep & Cook Time: 20 minutes
Macro Counts - Per Serving:
- Calories: 325
- Net Carbohydrates: 4 g
- Protein: 30 g
- Fat Content: 21 g

Ingredients:
- Ground beef (1 lb.)
- Salsa - ex. Pace Organic (.5 cup)
- Shredded cabbage (2 cups)
- Chili powder (2 tsp.)
- Shredded cheese (.75 cup)

Preparation Technique:
1. Brown the beef and drain the fat. Pour in the salsa, cabbage, and seasoning.
2. Cover and lower the heat. Simmer for 10 to 12 minutes using the medium heat temperature setting.
3. When the cabbage has softened, remove it from the heat and mix in the cheese.
4. Top it off using your favorite toppings, such as green onions or sour cream, and serve.

Chapter 8: Snacks & Appetizer Specialties

Smoothies

Avocado-Raspberry Smoothie

Servings Provided: 2
Prep & Cook Time: 5-6 minutes
Macro Counts - Per Serving:
- Calories: 227
- Net Carbohydrates: 4 g
- Protein: 2.5 g
- Fat Content: 20 g

Ingredients:
- Ripe avocado (1)
- Lemon juice (3 tbsp.)
- Water (1.33 cups)
- Frozen unsweetened raspberries/or choice of berries (.5 cup)
- Sugar equivalent - your preference (1 tbsp. + 1 tsp.)

Preparation Technique:
1. Chop the avocado into chunks.
2. Toss each of the fixings into a blender and mix until it's smooth.
3. Pour the smoothie into two glasses and serve.
4. Note: You can choose other berries, but be sure to calculate any additional carbs.

Blueberry Yogurt Smoothie

Servings Provided: 2
Prep & Cook Time: 5 minutes
Macro Counts - Per Serving:
- Calories: 70
- Net Carbohydrates: 2 g
- Protein: 2 g
- Fat Content: 5 g

Ingredients:
- Blueberries (10)
- Yogurt (.5 cup)
- Vanilla extract (.5 tsp.)
- Coconut milk (1 cup)
- Stevia (to taste)

Preparation Technique:
1. Add all of the fixings into the blender, mixing well.
2. When creamy, pour into two chilled mugs and enjoy.

Cinnamon Smoothie

Servings Provided: 1
Prep & Cook Time: 5 minutes
Macro Counts - Per Serving:
- Calories: 467
- Net Carbohydrates: 5 g
- Protein: 24 g
- Fat Content: 40 g

Ingredients:
- Coconut milk (.5 cup)
- Cinnamon (.5 tsp.)
- Water (.5 cup)
- Extra-virgin coconut oil or MCT oil (1 tbsp.)
- Ground chia seeds (1 tbsp.)
- Plain or vanilla whey protein (.25 cup)
- Optional: Stevia drops

Preparation Technique:
1. Pour the milk, cinnamon, protein powder, and chia seeds in a blender.
2. Empty the coconut oil, ice, and water. Add a few drops of stevia to your liking.

Strawberry Almond Smoothies

Servings Provided: 2
Prep & Cook Time: 5 minutes
Macro Counts - Per Serving:
- Calories: 304
- Net Carbohydrates: 7 g
- Protein: 15 g
- Fat Content: 25 g

Ingredients:
- Frozen unsweetened strawberries (.25 cup)
- Unsweetened almond milk (16 oz.)
- Heavy cream (.5 cup)
- Stevia (to your liking)
- Whey vanilla isolate powder (2 tbsp.)

Preparation Technique:
1. Measure and add all of the fixings into a blender.
2. Pulse the components until it's as you like it.

Delicious Snacks

Avocado & Bacon Caesar Deviled Eggs

Servings Provided: 1
Prep & Cook Time: 25 minutes
Macro Counts - Per Serving:
- Calories: 342
- Net Carbohydrates: 2 g
- Protein: 16 g
- Fat Content: 30 g

Ingredients:
- Eggs (2)
- Mayonnaise (1 tbsp.)
- Dijon mustard (.25 tsp.)
- Squeezed lemon (.125 tsp.)
- Garlic powder (.25 tsp.)
- Himalayan pink salt (.125 tsp.)
- Smoked paprika (.125 tsp.)
  Bacon-Avocado Filling
- Avocado (¼ of 1)
- Pastured bacon (1 slice

Preparation Technique:
  The Filling:
1. Chop and avocado and bacon into ¼-inch pieces.
2. Toss the bacon into a skillet, and cook using the medium heat setting for three minutes, or until browned.
3. Add the avocado and lower the temperature setting to low to simmer for an additional three minutes.

  The Eggs:
1. Pour two quarts of water into a pot to boil. Adjust the temperature setting to low. Gently add the eggs to cook for eight minutes.

2. Plunge the eggs into an ice water bath for three minutes. Once chilled, remove the peels and slice them in halves - lengthwise.
3. Gently transfer the yolks, the lemon, mayo, lemon, salt, mustard, and garlic powder into a food processor. Pulse the mixture until it's creamy smooth.
4. Spoon the filling into the egg white and dust with the paprika.

Bacon-Wrapped Brussel Sprouts

Servings Provided: 12
Prep & Cook Time: 45 minutes
Macro Counts - Per Serving:
- Calories: 58
- Net Carbohydrates: 1 g
- Fat Content: 4 g
- Protein: 4 g

Ingredients:
- Bacon (12 strips)
- Brussel sprouts (12 medium-large)
- Black pepper (to your liking)

Preparation Technique:
1. Set the oven temperature at 375° Fahrenheit. Prepare a baking tray with a layer of foil.
2. Rinse and dry the sprouts using a paper towel.
3. Place the sprout on a slice of bacon and roll it until covered. Arrange them on the baking tray and season to your liking.
4. Bake them for 30 to 35 minutes. Serve using a toothpick as a handle.

Cheese Quesadilla

Servings Provided: 1
Prep & Cook Time: 20 minutes
Macro Counts - Per Serving:
- Calories: 298.2
- Net Carbohydrates: 10.3 g
- Fat Content: 14.2 g
- Protein: 23 g

Ingredients:
- Low-carb/low-fat wraps -ex. Toufayan (13 g total carb & 8 g fiber)
- Mexican blend cheese ex. - Kraft shredded (.33 cup)
- Food Lion sour cream - full- fat (1 tbsp.)
- F.L. salsa (2 tbsp.)
- F.L. salted butter (about 1 tsp.)

Preparation Technique:
1. Lightly butter a wrapper and place it butter side down in griddle or skillet.
2. Add cheese - leaving about a ¼-inch edge.
3. Wait and cook until the cheese is mostly melted.
4. Close the quesadilla by folding in half, cooking until browned and crispy.
5. Flip it over and cook the other side the same way. Slice it into three wedges and serve with sour cream and a low-sugar keto-friendly salsa.
6. Note: Carbs counted used the specific brands listed; using other brands may change the counts.

Cobb Salad Bacon Cups

Servings Provided: 6
Prep & Cook Time: 1 hour 5 minutes
Macro Counts - Per Serving:
- Calories: 145
- Net Carbohydrates: 0.9 g
- Protein: 9.5 g
- Fat Content: 9.9 g

Ingredients:
- Thin-cut bacon (12 slices)
- Romaine lettuce (1 cup)
- Cooked chicken (.5 cup)
- California Avocado (half of 1)
- Hard-boiled egg (1)
- Tomato (.25 cup)
  Optional:
- Bleu cheese (2 tbsp.)
- Dressing of choice

Preparation Technique:
1. Finely chop the lettuce and slice the egg. Chop the chicken, tomato, and avocado. Crumble the cheese and set it aside.
2. Set the oven at 425° Fahrenheit. Cover the wells of a standard-sized muffin tin using a sheet of foil.
3. Slice six of the bacon slices in half and cover each cup with two halves - forming an x-type pattern (using the whole piece and secure it with a toothpick).
4. Bake them for about 35 minutes until the bacon is crunchy, and cool them for about 20 minutes. Remove the toothpicks and fill the cups.
5. Top it off with your favorite dressing (or not) and serve.

Roasted Salt & Pepper Radish Chips

Servings Provided: 4
Prep & Cook Time: 25 minutes
Macro Counts - Per Serving:
- Calories: 70
- Net Carbohydrates: 1.2 g
- Fat Content: 7.1 g
- Protein: 0.4 g

Ingredients:
- Fresh radishes (16 oz.)
- Melted coconut/olive oil (2 tbsp.)
- Black pepper and sea salt (.5 tsp. of each)

Preparation Technique:
1. Warm the oven to reach 400° Fahrenheit.
2. Use a mandolin to thinly slice the radishes. Place them in a container and toss them with the oil.
3. Layer them onto two baking trays, not overlapping, and dust with the pepper and salt.
4. Bake for 12 to 15 minutes and serve when ready.

Sweet Mustard Mini Sausages

Servings Provided: 4
Prep & Cook Time: 20 minutes
Macro Counts - Per Serving:
- Calories: 744
- Net Carbohydrates: 7.2 g
- Protein: 24 g
- Fat Content: 45 g

Ingredients:
- Swerve brown sugar (1 cup)
- Mustard powder (2 tsp.)
- Almond flour (3 tbsp.)
- White vinegar (.25 cup)
- Lemon juice (.25 cup)
- Tamari sauce (1 tsp.)
- Mini smoked sausages (2 lb.)

Preparation Technique:
1. Combine the mustard, flour, and swerve in a saucepan. Stir in the tamari sauce, vinegar, and juice.
2. Set the burner using the medium temperature setting. Once boiling, stir about two minutes until thickened.
3. Mix in the sausages and gently stir to cook for about five minutes.
4. Serve the delicious treat at any time.

Tasty Bacon & Cheese Balls

Servings Provided: 4
Prep & Cook Time: 25 minutes
Macro Counts - Per Serving:
- Calories: 538
- Net Carbohydrates: 0.5 g
- Fat Content: 50 g
- Protein: 22 g

Ingredients:
- Cream cheese (6 oz.)
- Sliced bacon (7 crumbled pieces)
- Gruyere shredded cheese (6 oz.)
- Unchilled butter (2 tbsp.)
- Red chili flakes (.5 tsp.)

Preparation Technique:
1. Fry the bacon in a skillet using the medium temperature setting until it's crispy (5 min.).
2. Pour the grease into a bowl and combine it with the rest of the fixings (chili flakes, butter, cream, and gruyere cheese). Pop it into the fridge to set (15 min.).
3. Remove the mixture and mold it into small walnut-sized balls, and roll in the crumbled bacon.
4. Serve any time!

Zucchini Nacho Chips

Servings Provided: 4
Prep & Cook Time: 35 minutes
Macro Counts - Per Serving:
- Calories: 66
- Net Carbohydrates: 1.6 g
- Fat Content: 6.9 g
- Protein: 0.6 g

Ingredients:
- Zucchini (1 large)
- Taco seasoning (1 tbsp.)
- Coconut oil (to fry)
- Salt (as needed)

Preparation Technique:
1. Use a mandolin to slice the zucchini. Place them over the sink in a colander and drizzle with salt. Wait five minutes and press out the water.
2. Prepare a pan or skillet (350° Fahrenheit) to heat the oil.
3. Add the zucchini (working in batches) or about 20 chips at a time.
4. Drain the grease on a paper towel-lined platter and serve with a sprinkle of the taco seasoning of choice.

Pizza Time

You can still enjoy a delicious pizza without all the additional carbs. Make our own crust and add the desired keto-friendly pizza toppings.

Cauliflower Pizza Crust

Servings Provided: 8
Prep & Cook Time: 45 minutes
Macro Counts - Per Serving:
- Calories: 106
- Net Carbohydrates: 3 g
- Protein: 10 g
- Fat Content: 6 g

Ingredients:
- Large egg (1)
- Cauliflower florets (1.5 cups)
- Grated parmesan cheese (1.5 cups)
  Optional Ingredients:
- Italian seasoning (.5 tbsp.)
- Garlic powder (.5 tbsp.)

Preparation Technique:
1. Set the oven temperature at 400° Fahrenheit.
2. Prepare a pizza pan or stone by lining it with a sheet of parchment paper.
3. Blitz the florets using a food processor to prepare the riced cauliflower. On the stovetop, sauté the florets for about 10 minutes or until softened.
4. Whisk the egg and blend in with the cheese and seasonings as desired.
5. Pour the rice into the mixture. Mix well and press with a spatula. (It's much easier to prepare two small pizzas.)
6. Spread the dough into the pan until it's about .25-inch thick. Bake until browned and firm (20 minutes).

7. Let the crust cool for a minimum of 5 to 10 minutes at
    room temperature. Add the chosen toppings. Bake until
    the cheese melts (5 to 10 minutes). Enjoy piping hot.

Crunchy Cheese Pizza with Mushrooms & Pepperoni

Servings Provided: 4
Prep & Cook Time: 15 minutes
Macro Counts - Per Serving:
- Calories: 298
- Net Carbohydrates: 1 g
- Protein: 19 g
- Fat Content: 23 g

Ingredients:
- Pepperoni (2 oz.)
- Mushrooms (3)
- Oregano (2 pinches - dried)
- Keto-friendly marinara sauce (2 tbsp.)
- Shredded cheddar cheese (.5 cup)
- Shredded mozzarella cheese (2 cups)
- Also Needed: High-heat non-stick skillet

Preparation Technique:
1. Thinly slice the pepperoni and mushrooms. Toss onto a lined cookie sheet. Broil/grill for three to five minutes.
2. Place the pizza pan on the grill using the high-temperature setting. Spread the mozzarella cheese evenly over the pan, then sprinkle using the cheddar. Work the cheese in - off the edges of the pan. Sprinkle with oregano.
3. Spread the marinara sauce around the melting cheese, trying not to work it down into the cheese - rather over it.
4. Add the pepperoni and mushrooms.
5. When the base is golden brown, crispy, and begins to lift as one piece, your pizza is ready.
6. Carefully slide the pizza onto a chopping board or cutting surface and slice into eight equal pieces before serving.

Healthy Veggie Pizza on Flourless Cauliflower Crust

Servings Provided: 8
Prep & Cook Time: 50 minutes
Macro Counts - Per Serving:
- Calories: 60
- Net Carbohydrates: 2.5 g
- Fat Content: 3.1 g
- Olive oil (2 tbsp.)

Ingredients:
- Cauliflower (1 cup)
- Low-fat mozzarella cheese (.75 cup - shredded)
- Egg (1)
- Crushed garlic (.5 tsp.)
- Dried oregano (1 tsp.)
- Pizza sauce (.5 cup)
- Mushrooms (.5 cup)
- Green bell pepper (half of 1)
- Red onion (half of 1)
- Vegetable oil spray (as needed)

Preparation Technique:
1. Set the oven to heat at 350° Fahrenheit.
2. Chop the mushrooms, onion, and bell pepper.
3. Shred the cauliflower in a food processor, and microwave it for eight minutes.
4. Mix in the egg, garlic, ½ cup of the cheese (save the rest for topping), and oregano.
5. Spray a pizza pan with a spritz of oil spray and spread with the cauliflower/cheese crust mixture.
6. Bake it for 10-15 minutes. Transfer the crust to the countertop and add the sauce, onion, mushrooms, bell pepper, and remaining cheese.
7. Pop the pan back in the oven for an additional 10-15 minutes to serve.

Vegetarian Spinach Keto Flatbread

Servings Provided: 6
Prep & Cook Time: 22-25 minutes
Macro Counts - Per Serving:
- Calories: 75
- Net Carbohydrates: 1 g
- Protein: 5 g
- Fat Content: 5 g

Ingredients:
- Shredded low-moisture mozzarella cheese (.75 cup)
- Cream cheese (1 tbsp.)
- Egg (1)
- Almond flour (2 tbsp.)
- Spinach (.25 cup)
- Garlic powder (.125 tsp.)
- Salt (to your liking)

Preparation Technique:
1. Set the oven temperature at 350° Fahrenheit.
2. Cook and drain the spinach.
3. Use a microwave-safe bowl to melt the cream cheese and mozzarella in the microwave using 30-second bursts, stirring in between intervals.
4. After the cheese is melted, mix in the almond flour, egg, and spinach.
5. Flatten the mixture on a parchment paper-lined baking sheet. Sprinkle using the garlic powder and salt.
6. Bake for 15 minutes. Flip the bread and bake for another five minutes.

Chapter 9: Dessert Specialties

Pudding Favorites

Avocado & Chocolate Pudding

Servings Provided: 2
Prep & Cook Time: 30 minutes
Macro Counts - Per Serving:
- Calories: 281
- Net Carbohydrates: 2 g
- Protein: 8 g
- Fat Content: 27 g

Ingredients:
- Cream cheese (2 oz.)
- Ripe medium avocado (1)
- Natural sweetener – swerve (1 tsp.)
- Vanilla extract (.25 tsp.)
- Unsweetened cocoa powder (4 tbsp.)
- Pink salt (1 pinch)

Preparation Technique:
1. Combine the cream cheese with the avocado, sweetener, vanilla, cocoa powder, and salt into the blender or processor.
2. Pulse until creamy smooth.
3. Measure into fancy dessert dishes and chill for at least ½ hour.

Cheesecake Pudding

Servings Provided: 4
Prep & Cook Time: 10 minutes (+) chill time
Macro Counts - Per Serving:
- Calories: 356
- Net Carbohydrates: 5 g
- Protein: 5 g
- Fat Content: 36 g

Ingredients:
- Cream cheese or Neufchatel cheese (1 block)
- Heavy whipping cream (.5 cup)
- Lemon juice (1 tsp.)
- Sour cream (.5 cup)
- Liquid stevia (20 drops)
- Vanilla extract (1 tsp.)

Preparation Technique:
1. Microwave the cream cheese for 30 seconds or leave on the counter to soften for a few minutes before using.
2. Whip the sour cream and whipping cream together with the mixer until soft peaks form. Combine with the rest of the fixings and whip until fluffy.
3. Portion into four dishes to chill. Place a layer of the wrap over the dish and store in the fridge.
4. When ready to eat, garnish with some berries if you like.
5. Note: If you add berries, be sure to add the carbs.

Delicious Cakes

Carrot Almond Cake

Servings Provided: 8
Prep & Cook Time: 1 hour
Macro Counts - Per Serving:
- Calories: 268
- Net Carbohydrates: 4 g
- Fat Content: 25 g
- Protein: 6 g

Ingredients:
- Eggs (3)
- Apple pie spice (1.5 tsp.)
- Almond flour (1 cup)
- Swerve (.66 cup)
- Baking powder (1 tsp.)
- Coconut oil (.25 cup)
- Shredded carrots (1 cup)
- Heavy whipping cream (.5 cup)
- Chopped walnuts (.5 cup)

Preparation Technique:
1. Grease the cake pan. Combine all of the fixings with the mixer until well mixed. Pour the mix into the pan and cover with a layer of foil.
2. Pour two cups of water into the Instant Pot bowl along with the steamer rack.
3. Arrange the pan on the trivet and set the pot using the cake button (40 min.).
4. Natural-release the pressure for ten minutes. Then, quick-release the rest of the built-up steam pressure.
5. Place on a rack to cool before frosting or serve it plain.

Chocolate Lava Cake

Servings Provided: 4
Prep & Cook Time: 35-40 minutes
Macro Counts - Per Serving:
- Calories: 189
- Net Carbohydrates: 3 g
- Protein: 8 g
- Fat Content: 17 g

Ingredients:
- Unsweetened cocoa powder (.5 cup)
- Melted butter (.25 cup)
- Eggs (4)
- Sugar-free chocolate sauce (.25 cup)
- Sea salt (.5 tsp.)
- Ground cinnamon (.5 tsp.)
- Pure vanilla extract (1 tsp.)
- Stevia (.25 cup)
- Also Needed: Ice cube tray & 4 ramekins

Preparation Technique:
1. Pour one tablespoon of the chocolate sauce into four of the tray slots and freeze.
2. Warm up the oven to 350° Fahrenheit. Lightly grease the ramekins with butter or a spritz of oil.
3. Mix the salt, cinnamon, cocoa powder, and stevia until combined. Whisk in the eggs – one at a time. Stir in the melted vanilla extract and butter.
4. Fill each of the ramekins halfway and add one of the frozen chocolates. Cover the rest of the container with the cake batter.
5. Bake for 13-14 minutes. When they're set, place on a wire rack to cool for about five minutes. Remove and put on a serving dish.
6. Enjoy by slicing its molten center.

Glazed Pound Cake

Servings Provided: 16
Prep & Cook Time: 2 hours
Macro Counts - Per Serving:
- Calories: 254
- Net Carbohydrates: 2.5 g
- Protein: 7.9 g
- Fat Content: 23.4 g

Ingredients:
- Salt (.5 tsp.)
- Almond flour (2.5 cups)
- Softened - unsalted butter (.5 cup)
- Erythritol (1.5 cups)
- Unchilled eggs (8)
- Lemon extract (.5 tsp.)
- Vanilla extract (1.5 tsp.)
- Cream cheese (8 oz.)
- Baking powder (1.5 tsp.)
  The Glaze:
- Powdered erythritol (.25 cup)
- Heavy whipping cream (3 tbsp.)
- Vanilla extract (.5 tsp.)

Preparation Technique:
1. Warm the oven to 350° Fahrenheit.
2. Whisk the baking powder, almond flour, and salt. Set aside.
3. Cream the erythritol, butter, and softened cream cheese chunks. Mix until smooth in a large mixing container.
4. Whisk and add the eggs with the lemon and vanilla extract. Blend with the rest of the fixings using a hand mixer until smooth.
5. Dump the batter into a loaf pan. Bake for one to two hours.
6. Prepare a glaze. Mix in the vanilla extract, powdered erythritol, and heavy whipping cream until smooth.

7. You must let the cake cool completely before adding the
    glaze.

Lemon Cake

Servings Provided: 8
Prep & Cook Time: 3.5 hours
Macro Counts - Per Serving:
- Calories: 350
- Net Carbohydrates: 5.2 g
- Protein: 7.6 g
- Fat Content: 33 g

Ingredients:
- Coconut flour (.5 cup)
- Baking powder (2 tsp.)
- Almond flour (1.5 cups)
- Swerve (or) Pyure A-P (3 tbsp.)
- Optional: Xanthan gum (.5 tsp.)
- Whipping cream (.5 cup)
- Melted butter (.5 cup)
- Zest & juice (2 lemons)
- Eggs (2)
     Ingredients for the Topping:
- Pyure all-purpose/Swerve (3 tbsp.)
- Lemon juice (2 tbsp.)
- Boiling water (.5 cup)
- Melted butter (2 tbsp.)
- Suggested: 2-4-quart slow cooker

Preparation Technique:
1. For the Cake: Mix the dry ingredients in a container. Whisk the egg with the lemon juice and zest, butter, and whipping cream. Whisk all of the fixings and scoop out the dough into the prepared slow cooker.
2. For the Topping: Mix all of the topping ingredients in a container and empty over the batter in the cooker.
3. Place the lid on the cooker for two to three hours on the high setting.
4. Serve warm with some fresh fruit or whipped cream.

Spice Cakes

Servings Provided: 12
Prep & Cook Time: 25 minutes
Macro Counts - Per Serving:
- Calories: 277
- Net Carbohydrates: 3 g
- Protein: 6 g
- Fat Content: 27 g

Ingredients:
- Salted butter (.5 cup)
- Erythritol (.75 cup)
- Eggs (4 - divided)
- Vanilla extract (1 tsp.)
- Ground cloves (.25 tsp.)
- Baking powder (2 tsp.)
- Allspice (.5 tsp.)
- Nutmeg (.5 tsp.
- Almond flour (2 cups)
- Cinnamon (.5 tsp.)
- Ginger (.5 tsp.)
- Water (5 tbsp.)
- Also Needed: Cupcake tray

Preparation Technique:
1. Warm the oven temperature to 350° Fahrenheit. Prepare the baking tray with liners (12).
2. Mix the butter and erythritol with a hand mixer. Once it's smooth, combine with two eggs and the vanilla. Add the rest of the eggs and mix well.
3. Grind the clove to a fine powder and add with the rest of the spices. Whisk into the mixture. Stir in the baking powder and almond flour. Blend in the water. When the batter is smooth, add to the prepared tin.
4. Bake for 15 minutes. Enjoy any time.

Vanilla - Sour Cream Cupcakes

Servings Provided: 12
Prep & Cook Time: 45 minutes
Macro Counts - Per Serving:
- Calories: 128
- Net Carbohydrates: 2 g
- Fat Content: 11 g
- Protein: 4 g

Ingredients:
- Butter (4 tbsp.)
- Swerve or your favorite sweetener (1.5 cups)
- Salt (.25 tsp.)
- Eggs (4)
- Sour cream (.25 cup)
- Vanilla (1 tsp.)
- Almond flour (1 cup)
- Baking powder (1 tsp.)
- Coconut flour (.25 cup)

Preparation Technique:
1. Warm the oven at 350° Fahrenheit.
2. Prepare the butter and sweetener until creamy and fluffy using the mixer.
3. Blend in the vanilla and sour cream. Mix well.
4. One at a time, fold in the eggs.
5. Sift and blend in both types of flour, salt, and baking powder.
6. Divide the batter between the cups.
7. Bake for 20 to 25 minutes. Times may vary according to your oven hotness.
8. Cool completely and place in the fridge for fresher results.

Bar Cakes & Cookies

Browned Butter Chocolate Chip Blondies

Servings Provided: 16
Prep & Cook Time: 35 minutes
Macro Counts - Per Serving:
- Calories: 161
- Net Carbohydrates: 3 g
- Protein: 3.8 g
- Fat Content: 14.4 g

Ingredients:
- Butter (.5 cup)
- Almond flour (2 cups)
- Swerve sweetener (.25 cup)
- Baking powder (1 tsp.)
- Salt (.5 tsp.)
- Sukrin Gold (.25 cup) *or* more swerve + molasses (2 tsp.)
- Large egg (1)
- Sugar-free chocolate chips (.33 cup)
- Vanilla extract (.5 tsp.)
- Also Needed: 9x9-inch baking pan

Preparation Technique:
1. Set the oven temperature at 325° Fahrenheit. Lightly grease the pan.
2. Toss the butter into the pan using the medium temperature setting. Cook until the butter is melted and becomes a deep amber (4-5 min.).
3. Remove the pan from the burner to cool.
4. Whisk the almond flour with the salt, baking powder, and sweeteners.
5. Whisk the egg and add it to the mixture with the browned butter and vanilla extract until thoroughly combined. Fold in the chocolate chips.

6. Evenly press the dough into the prepared pan.
7. Set a timer to bake for 15-20 minutes or until just set and golden brown.
8. Let the blondies cool in the pan. Slice into squares and serve as desired.

Chocolate Chip Cookies

Servings Provided: 18
Prep & Cook Time: 30 minutes
Macro Counts - Per Serving:
- Calories: 96
- Net Carbohydrates: 1 g
- Protein: 2 g
- Fat Content: 9 g

Ingredients:
- Eggs (2 large)
- Grass-fed melted butter (1 stick - .5 cup)
- Pure vanilla extract - alcohol-free (2 tsp.)
- Heavy cream (2 tbsp.)
- Almond flour (2.75 cups)
- Kosher salt (.25 tsp.)
- Swerve (.5 cup or to taste)
- Dark chocolate chips - ex. Lily's (.75 cup)
- Cooking spray - as needed

Preparation Technique:
1. Set the oven temperature at 350° Fahrenheit. Prepare the pan.
2. Whisk the egg with the heavy cream, butter, vanilla, almond flour, salt, and swerve.
3. Fold the chocolate chips into the batter.
4. Form the mixture into one-inch balls. Flatten the balls with the glass or your hands that's been lightly greased with cooking spray.
5. Arrange the cookies about three inches apart on the cookie sheets.
6. Bake until the cookies are golden, about 17-19 minutes.

Key Lime Bars

Servings Provided: 16
Prep & Cook Time: 50 minutes + chilling time (1 hr.)
Macro Counts - Per Serving:
- Calories: 188
- Net Carbohydrates: 2.4 g
- Protein: 3.4 g
- Fat Content: 17.5 g

Ingredients:
The Crust:
- Almond flour (1.25 cups)
- Swerve Sweetener (.33 cup)
- Salt (.25 tsp.)
- Melted butter (.25 cup)
The Filling:
- Unchilled cream cheese (3 oz. - softened)
- Lime zest (2 tsp.)
- Sugar-free condensed milk (1 cup)
- Egg yolks (4)
- Key lime juice (6 tbsp.)
- Also Suggested: 8x8-inch baking pan

Preparation Technique - The Crust:
1. Warm the oven to 325° Fahrenheit.
2. Whisk the almond flour with the salt and sweetener.
3. Melt the butter and add to the mixture to make the batter.
4. Pour the batter into the pan. Press firmly into the bottom.
5. Bake until just golden brown around the edges (for 12-15 min.).
6. Transfer to the countertop to cool.

Preparation Technique - The Key Lime:
1. Beat the cream cheese and lime zest until creamy smooth.
2. Whisk and fold in the egg yolks until well mixed.

3. Slowly pour in the juice from the lime and condensed milk. Stir until the filling is creamy smooth.
4. Add the filling into the crust. Bake it for 15-20 minutes.
5. Remove and cool. Store in the fridge for at least one hour to set.
6. Top with lightly sweetened whipped cream and lime slices if desired.

Raspberry Fudge

Servings Provided: 12
Preparation & Cook Time: 2 hours 15 minutes
Macro Counts - Per Serving:
- Calories: 242
- Net Carbohydrates: 4.4 g
- Protein: 2.6 g
- Fat Content: 25.3 g

Ingredients:
- Cream cheese (16 oz.)
- Butter (1 cup)
- White sugar substitute (.25 cup)
- Unsweetened cocoa powder (6 tbsp.)
- Heavy cream (2 tbsp.)
- Vanilla extract (2 tsp.)
- Raspberry extract (1 tsp.)
- Chopped walnuts (.33 cup)

Preparation Technique:
1. Take the cream cheese and butter out of the fridge ahead of time until it reaches room temperature.
2. Mix the cream cheese and butter in the mixing bowl with the mixer.
3. When smooth, mix with the rest of the fixings until well incorporated.
4. Microwave using the high setting for 30 seconds. Blend with the mixer again until smooth.
5. Empty into the prepared pan (1-inch layer). Cover the pan and chill for at least two hours in the fridge.
6. Slice into 12 portions.
7. Serve and enjoy or store in the fridge for a delicious treat later.

Sunflower Seed Surprise Cookies

Servings Provided: 12
Prep & Cook Time: 20 minutes
Macro Counts - Per Serving:
- Calories: 69
- Net Carbohydrates: 0.64 g
- Protein: 2.3 g
- Fat Content: 6.3 g

Ingredients:
- Egg (50 g/1 large egg)
- Sugar-free sunflower seed butter (100 g/.75 cup)
- Coconut oil (16 g/1 rounded tbsp.)
- Optional: Truvia (12 g/1 tbsp.)
- Vanilla extract (2 g/.5 tsp.)
- Salt - Baking powder & soda (1 g/1 pinch each)

Preparation Technique:
1. Warm the oven temperature setting to 350° Fahrenheit. Set the rack in the upper portion of the oven.
2. Prepare a cookie tray using a layer of parchment baking paper.
3. Mix all of the fixings in a large container.
4. Roll and flatten the mixture into 12 balls about the width of a quarter.
5. Bake the cookies for seven to nine minutes until they're firm in the center.
6. Cool the cookies for a couple of hours.

Pies & Cheesecakes

Keto Pie Crust

Servings Provided: 10
Prep & Cook Time: varies - 20-30 minutes
Macro Counts - Per Serving:
- Net Carbohydrates: 1.8 g
- Calories: 187
- Fat Content: 12.7 g
- Protein: 3.7 g

Ingredients:
- Salt (.25 tsp.)
- Butter - melted (.25 cup)

Preparation Technique:
1. Whisk the salt, sweetener, and flour in a mixing container. Fold in the melted butter to form coarse crumbs.
2. Dump it into a pie plate and press it firmly to the sides and bottom. Prick it using a toothpick or fork.
3. For unfilled Crust: Bake 325° Fahrenheit for about 20 minutes.
4. For filled Crust: Pre-bake it for 10-12 minutes before adding the fixings. Cover the edges to avoid over-browning.

Delicious Cheesecake

Servings Provided: 12
Prep & Cook Time: 52 minutes
Macro Counts - Per Serving:
- Calories: 231.8
- Net Carbohydrates: 3.4 g
- Protein: 4.9 g
- Fat Content: 22.3 g

Ingredients:
- Eggs (2)
- Vanilla extract (2 tsp.)
- Sour cream (1.5 cups)
- Splenda granules/another keto-friendly sweetener (.5 cup)
- Unchilled cream cheese (16 oz.)
- Melted butter (2 tbsp.)
- Also Needed: 12 ramekins or 10-inch springform pan

Preparation Technique:
1. Warm the oven temperature at 350° Fahrenheit.
2. Whisk the eggs, vanilla, sour cream, and Splenda in a large mixing container. Work in the cream cheese and butter.
3. Spoon and combine about ½ cup of the mixture into another bowl and add the raspberry flavoring.
4. Spoon the rest of the mix into the chosen container.
5. Scoop a spoon of the raspberry batter over the top. Swirl it through the plain mixture.
6. Prepare a crust from ¼ cup of Splenda, ¼ cup of butter, and 1 ½ cups ground almonds. Mix it like a graham cracker crust and add it to the ramekins/pan.
7. Arrange the ramekins in a water bath (a shallow pan with water) in the oven below the ramekins/pan.
8. Bake for 20-25 minutes for ramekins or 35-40 minutes in a springform pan. The cake will firm up when refrigerated.
9. Top it off using raspberries and whipped cream - but add the carbs. Freeze if desired.

10. *Note*: The nutritional calculations do not include crust.

Low-Carb Chocolate Cheesecake

Servings Provided: 12
Prep & Cook Time: 55 minutes
Macro Counts - Per Serving:
- Calories: 207.7
- Net Carbohydrates: 4.7 g
- Protein: 4.8 g
- Fat Content: 20 g

Ingredients:
- Cream cheese (.5 cup)
- Heavy cream (16 oz.)
- Sugar-Free Chocolate Instant Pudding mix (1 pkg.)
- Splenda stevia natural (.5 cup - reserve 3 tbsp. for sauce)
- Vanilla extract (1 tsp.)
- Eggs (2)
  The Sauce:
- Butter (2 tbsp.)
- Cocoa (4 tbsp.)
- Splenda (3 tbsp.)

Preparation Technique:
1. Prepare the sauce. Use a microwave or stovetop to melt the butter, cocoa, and Splenda. Drizzle the sauce over the cake after it comes out of the oven. Set it to the side.
2. Prep the cake. Mix the cream cheese, vanilla, Splenda, and eggs. Set aside.
3. Combine the cream and pudding in another mixing container and add it to the cream cheese mixture using the high blender setting until thoroughly mixed.
4. Lightly spritz a pie plate and a cooking oil spray.
5. Scoop the cheesecake mixture into the pan. Bake uncovered at 350° Fahrenheit for 35 to 40 minutes. Remove from the oven and drizzle the chocolate mixture over top.
6. Refrigerate and serve chilled.

Fat Bombs

Carrot Cake Fat Bombs

Servings Provided: 45 bombs
Prep & Cook Time: 1 hour 15 minutes
Macro Counts - Per Serving:
- Calories: 80.27
- Net Carbohydrates: 0.86 g
- Protein: 1.12 g
- Fat Content: 8.04 g

Ingredients:
- Grated carrots (100 g/0.75 cup)
- Melted coconut manna (224 g/1 cup)
- Unchilled - salted butter (114 g/0.5 cup)
- Unchilled cream cheese (114 g/0.5 cup)
- Flax meal (28 g/2 tbsp.)
- Chopped walnuts (117 g/1 cup)
- Cinnamon (5 g/2 tsp.)
- Optional: Truvia (1 packet) or liquid stevia (as desired)

Preparation Technique:
1. Grate and add the carrots, coconut manna, cream cheese, butter, sweetener (if using), and flax meal in a food processor. Pulse until the fixings are thoroughly combined.
2. If the mixture is too soft to roll into balls, pop it into the fridge until it can easily be handled.
3. Meanwhile, prepare a baking tray with a layer of waxed or parchment baking paper. Roll the dough batch into 45 one-inch balls and place them in a single layer in the pan.
4. Sprinkle them using the walnuts and cinnamon. Using the edges of the paper, toss until they are evenly coated. Gently

press the coating into the bites and store the finished fat bombs in an airtight container in the refrigerator.

Pumpkin Spice Fat Bombs

Servings Provided: 24
Prep & Cook Time: 16 minutes
Macro Counts - Per Serving:
- Calories: 66
- Net Carbohydrates: 0.5 g
- Fat Content: 7 g
- Protein: 0.4 g

Ingredients:
- Unchilled butter (.5 cup/114 g)
- Unsweetened pumpkin puree (.25 cup/60g)
- Coconut butter - melted but not hot (.5 cup/114 g)
- Cinnamon/combination of spices - ex. - cloves, allspice, nutmeg, etc. (1 tsp./3 g)

Preparation Technique:
1. Toss all of the fixings into a mixing container and mix until smooth.
2. Scoop the batter into silicone molds and taping them gently to remove air bubbles.
3. Freeze and enjoy once they are solid.

Strawberry Ginger Fat Bomb

Servings Provided: 28
Prep & Cook Time: 30 minutes
Macro Counts - Per Serving:
- Calories: 97
- Net Carbohydrates: 0.8 g
- Fat Content: 10 g
- Protein: 0.7 g

Ingredients:
- Coconut oil (120 g)
- Coconut manna (120 g)
- Macadamia nuts - dry roasted with salt (120 g)
- Fresh ginger (10 g)
- Fresh strawberries (120 g)
- Black pepper (1 pinch)

Preparation Technique:
1. Melt the coconut manna and oil in a glass bowl. (Use an electric mug warmer if you have one.)
2. Toss all of the fixings into a food processor fitted with a chopping blade. Puree until smooth.
3. Enjoy it - as is or freeze in a silicone mold, so the fat bombs will last much longer.

Chapter 10: Your 21-Day Meal Plan

You will find this meal plan very successful for assisting in your weight loss plans as you approach or pass the age of 50. Each one is compiled leaving you plenty of room to add extra healthy fruits or snacks. The net carbs have been calculated for your convenience, so they can be easily switched if you don't want to prepare the meals as suggested. Please enjoy each one!

Day 1: 16.7 Total Net Carbs

Breakfast: Best Scrambled Eggs - 2.9 g

Lunch: Buffalo Chicken Soup - 4 g

Dinner: Crab Cakes - 4 g & Creamy Spinach-Rich Ballet - 2.9 g

Dessert: Key Lime Bars - 2.4 g

Optional Snack: Pumpkin Spice Fat Bombs - 0.5 g

Day 2: 16.4 Total Net Carbs

Breakfast: Blueberry Muffins - 5 g

Lunch: Snap Pea & Scallion Salad - Hot - 3 g

Dinner: Maple Country-Style Pork Ribs - Slow-Cooked - 2 g

Dessert: Raspberry Fudge - 4.4 g

Optional Snack: Avocado & Bacon Caesar Deviled Eggs - 2 g

Day 3: 18.16 Total Net Carbs

Breakfast: Ham & Egg Cups - 0.96 g

Lunch: Cauliflower & Kielbasa Soup - 5.7 g

Dinner: Parmesan Chicken - 0.4 g &

Creamy Green Cabbage - 8.2 g

Dessert: Leftover Key Lime Bars - 2.4 g

Optional Snack: Tasty Bacon & Cheese Balls - 0.5 g

Day 4: 20.5 Total Net Carbs

Breakfast: Flaxseed Porridge - 4 g

Lunch: Healthy Veggie Pizza on Flourless Cauliflower Crust - 2.5 g

Dinner: Parmesan Shrimp - 4.5 & Red Pepper Zoodles - 4.1 g

Dessert: Leftover Raspberry Fudge - 4.4 g

Optional Snack: Bacon-Wrapped Brussel Sprouts - 1 g

Day 5: 14.39 Total Net Carbs

Breakfast: Scrambled Eggs with Mayo - 0.99 g

Lunch: Italian Sausage Soup With Tomatoes & Zucchini Noodles - 4 g

Dinner: Asian-Inspired Pork Chops - 5.5 g

Dessert: Browned Butter Chocolate Chip Blondies - 3 g

Optional Snack: Cobb Salad Bacon Cups - 0.9 g

Day 6: 11.7 Total Net Carbs

Breakfast: Macadamia Keto Pancakes - 1.5 g

Lunch: Cauliflower Beef Curry - 3 g

Dinner: Mediterranean Grilled Ahi Tuna - 0.4 g &

Mushroom & Cauliflower Risotto - 4.3 g

Dessert: Vanilla - Sour Cream Cupcakes - 2 g

Optional Snack: Tasty Bacon & Cheese Balls - 0.5 g

Day 7: 14.5 Total Net Carbs

Breakfast: Sausage Egg Casserole - 2.1 g

Lunch: Spinach - Broccoli - Feta Salad - 4.9 g

Dinner: Lamb & Asparagus with Tangy Sauce - 3.7 g

Dessert: Leftover Browned Butter Chocolate Chip Blondies - 3 g

Optional Snack: Strawberry Ginger Fat Bomb - 0.8 g

Day 8: 20.2 Total Net Carbs

Breakfast: Old-Fashioned Baked Custard - Heavy Cream - 3 g

Lunch: Creamy Chicken Broccoli - 5 g

Dinner: BBQ Flank Steak - 1 g

Dessert: Carrot Almond Cake - 4 g

Optional Snack: Sweet Mustard Mini Sausages - 7.2 g

Day 9: 16.5 Total Net Carbs

Breakfast: Egg Muffins - 1 g

Lunch: Colby Cauliflower Soup & Pancetta Chips - 6 g

Dinner: Parmesan Shrimp - 4.5

Dessert: Leftover Carrot Almond Cake - 4 g

Optional Snack: Avocado Tuna Melt Bites - 1 g

Day 10: 12.34 Total Net Carbs

Breakfast: Cauliflower & Cheddar Hash Browns - 2.5 g

Lunch: Cabbage Patties - 1 g

Dinner: Balsamic Grilled Chicken Breast - 2.6 g &

Stuffed Mushrooms - 2.6 g

Dessert: Spice Cakes - 3 g

Optional Snack: Sunflower Seed Surprise Cookies - 0.64 g

Day 11: 19.1 Total Net Carbs

Breakfast: Baked Custard - Dairy-Free - 3 g

Lunch: Chicken Nuggets - 11 g

Dinner: Roasted Leg Of Lamb - 1 g

Dessert: Leftover Spice Cakes - 3 g

Optional Snack: Dried Beef & Cream Cheese Ball - 1.1 g

Day 12: 15.36 Total Net Carbs

Breakfast: Bacon & Egg Fat Bombs - 0.2 g

Lunch: Creamy Taco Soup - 4 g

Dinner: Crockpot Pork Chops - 7.7 g

Dessert: Chocolate Lava Cake - 3 g

Optional Snack: Sunflower Seed Surprise Cookies - 0.64 g

Day 13: 13.9 Total Net Carbs

Breakfast: Crispy Light Waffles - 1 g

Lunch: Zucchini Noodle Gratin - 3 g

Dinner: Parmesan Crusted Tilapia - 0.2 g

Dessert: Low-Carb Chocolate Cheesecake - 4.7 g

Optional Snack: Cinnamon Smoothie - 5 g

Day 14: 16.4 Total Net Carbs

Breakfast: Cream Cheese Eggs - 3 g

Lunch: Cool & Spicy Jicama Slaw - 3 g

Dinner: Shrimp Scampi For Garlic Lovers - 1.2 g

Dessert: Lemon Cake - 5.2 g

Optional Snack: Avocado-Raspberry Smoothie - 4 g

Day 15: 21 Total Net Carbs

Breakfast: Hot Pockets - 2 g

Lunch: Chicken Zoodle Soup - 4 g

Dinner: Hot Tex-Mex Pork Casserole - 7.8 g

Dessert: Leftover Lemon Cake - 5.2 g

Optional Snack: Blueberry Yogurt Smoothie - 2 g

Day 16: 18.3 Total Net Carbs

Breakfast: Bacon & Brie Frittata - 1.7 g

Lunch: Citrus Cauliflower Salad - 1 g

Dinner: Salmon Cakes - 3.6 g

Dessert: Cheesecake Pudding - 5 g

Optional Snack: Strawberry Almond Smoothies - 7 g

Day 17: 19.16 Total Net Carbs

Breakfast: Sausage Gravy & Biscuits - 2 g

Lunch: Cheese Quesadilla - 10.3 g

Dinner: Balsamic Grilled Chicken Breast - 2.6 g

Dessert: Delicious Cheesecake - 3.4 g

Optional Snack: Carrot Cake Fat Bombs - 0.86 g

Day 18: 19 Total Net Carbs

Breakfast: BLT Brunch Wrap - 2 g

Lunch: Crunchy Fish & Chaffle Bites - 1.3 g

Dinner: Garlic & Olive Oil Spaghetti Squash - 11.6 g

Dessert: Glazed Pound Cake - 2.5 g

Optional Snack: Zucchini Nacho Chips - 1.6 g

Day 19: 15.64 Total Net Carbs

Breakfast: Pigs in Pancakes - 3.04 g

Lunch: Kofta Kebab - 1 g

Dinner: Mississippi Pot Roast - 3 g & Marinara Zoodles - 5.1 g

Dessert: Leftover Glazed Pound Cake - 2.5 g

Optional Snack: Chocolate Chip Cookies - 1 g

Day 20: 12 Total Net Carbs

Breakfast: Ham & Spinach Mini Quiche - 2 g

Lunch: Rainbow Salad - 1 g

Dinner: Quick & Easy Creamy Mushroom Chicken - 5.8 g

Dessert: Avocado & Chocolate Pudding - 2 g

Optional Snack: Roasted Salt & Pepper Radish Chips - 1.2 g

Day 21: 12.6 Total Net Carbs

Breakfast: Southwestern Cauliflower Breakfast Pizza - 2.6 g

Lunch: Shirataki Soup - 1.5 g

Dinner: Fiesta Lime Chicken - 5.6 g

Dessert: Shrimp Scampi - 1.9 g

Optional Snack: Chocolate Chip Cookies - 1 g

You now have the map, but do you know how to resist the urge to splurge in a non-keto option? Let's see how it works!

- *Sugary Foods*: Several things can trigger the desire for sugar, but typically phosphorous, and tryptophan are the culprits. Have a portion of cheese, cauliflower, or broccoli.

- *Fatty or Oily Foods:* The levels of calcium and chloride need repair with some spinach, broccoli, or cheese.

- *Salty Foods*: Your body is craving silicon. Have a few nuts and seeds; just be sure to count them into your daily counts.

- *Chocolate*: The carbon, magnesium, and chromium levels are requesting a portion of spinach, nuts, and seeds, or some broccoli and cheese.

As you prepare your list of favorites; consider the process of meal prep. Be prepared when family and friends stop by for an unexpected visit. These are a few suggestions to get you started.

Save tons of time and money and learn how to prep so you always have fresh foods to match your vegetarian dishes. You're going to need plastic wrap, tin foil, wax paper, and lots of food storage containers. The best ones are clear, so when they're stacked in the fridge; you can tell what the contents are without any guesswork. Mason jars are also an excellent choice and a lot of fun for salads; you can layer different colored vegetables in them and then just add dressing and shake.

Buy vegetables in bulk or when in season and freeze them. As an example, avocados can be expensive, but if you come across some that are discounted because they're about to be past their sell-by date, you can buy them and freeze the flesh to use in smoothies.

Roast the Vegetables: By roasting veggies, you are not only able to quickly prepare them bulk, but you can also roast them on the same pan with a layer of tin foil. It is a good idea to prepare three or four different veggies for one week, so you have a variety to go along with your new keto diet plan.

Purchase & Prepare Eggs: You can hard-boil the eggs to last for a week and store them in the refrigerator. The simplest way to know when you made them is to store them in the original container. Leave the shells on and mark the carton with the date and time. You can also use them in sandwiches or with a salad – anytime!

The reason to refrain from peeling the eggs is that they can absorb and create smells and mix flavors in the fridge. You don't want that to happen - so be sure the container used is airtight. Just place the whole carton into a zipper type bag for safe and easy access.

Choose Fresh Berries: Many berries are notorious for spoiling easily. Don't worry there's an easy way to keep them fresh all week. Add three cups of water to one cup of vinegar in a large mixing container. Soak the berries in the mixture for about five minutes. Drain and pat them until they're as dry as you can get them. Store them in an airtight container lined with paper towels. Leave a crack the lid open to keep letting moisture escape.

Choose blueberries and strawberries over blackberries or raspberries. To prevent bruising, attempt to keep them in a single layer rather than piling them on top of each other. For example, Tupperware makes a bacon container and other items that would be ideal.

Bulk Prep The Carbs. Make a large pot of lentils, beans, or quinoa; then, you can either divide it into two or three different flavors with your herbs and spices or space it out over your containers and add a sauce to finish it off.
These are just a few of the ways to enjoy your lifestyle changes using the ketogenic dieting methods. Have some fun, and get started!

Chapter 11: A Final Word – Exercise

You have taken all the right steps! You have purchased the ketogenic diet plan with a 21-day meal plan. You have a bunch of new recipes to try! All that is left is a trip to the market and a new motivation, beginning in the exercise department. Just because you are over 50 doesn't mean you don't need to stay in shape! Try some of these super ways to get going!

The best drive for you is to attain your goals is - slowly - step-by-step. As you reach the first set of goals, ease into the next phase - moving forward to the next one. You'll be climbing the mountain top in small stages versus the ideals of trying to lose ten pounds in one day. Make the process simple and stick with it for a couple of weeks. Guess what, you can do it!

If you have grandchildren or other children in your life. Exercise your spirit, mind, and body. Run around with the kids for a beautiful-heartfelt workout. If you don't believe it, give it a day! You will be tired - yet rewarded with love and a bunch of lost calories. Look at the fun, and the kids are entertained.

Suppose you want to get active without it feeling like a workout. In that case, regular gardening has the benefit of providing you with the fresh air and upping your Vitamin D. You will also provide a beautiful garden.

If you love being outside instead of in a gym, then a brisk stroll or run around your local park or neighborhood is the thing for you.

Grab a friend or a neighbor - anyone - who could benefit from a bit of exercise. Be each other's support and motivator as you work harder and burn more calories.

Get Motivated Using Balance Exercises

As you get older, you may not be as steady on your feet. Don't be discouraged; there are a few simple exercises you can perform in just a few minutes. It will bring back motivation once you realize you still have the opportunity to improve your gait.

All you need is the kitchen countertop or a steady chair for support. Let's give it a try!

- *Step 1: Try the Parallel Stance*: Relax and take a few deep breaths. Stand and extend your feet apart (about a hip's width). Do not hold onto the chair (it's there for back-up), and keep the stance for ten seconds. If you did not wobble during that time, try step 2.

- *Step 2: Try the Semi-Tandem Stance*: Take a cleansing breath as you place one foot halfway in front of the other. Hold the pose for ten seconds - not holding a chair. It is similar to the stance used by an officer for a sobriety check. If you are a success, try the last pose.

- *Step 3: Try the Tandem Stance*: Take in a breath of fresh air. Place your mind in the tone that you are on a tightrope. Take the position (holding the chair for support if needed), standing with one foot directly in front of the other, and keep the pose for ten seconds. Slowly eliminate contact with a chair.

If you believe you are in good physical health, strength training is a crucial exercise that's important as we get older. It can help maintain muscle mass. Consider a bit of weight training with a set of light dumbbells.

There are plenty of other options that don't require any equipment which can easily be done at home. Don't worry if you're not sure how to get started.

Walking

Many older folks set a goal of 10,000 steps daily. Don't just shuffle around the house. Put on a supportive pair of walking shoes and go for a brisk walk. You will be surprised how you can clear your mind on a peaceful walk. Put in the earbuds and turn on the tunes.

If you have a dog, go for a walk with your favorite pal. Your pet will enjoy it, and it will allow you to do it for the well-being of your dog. Take a slightly longer walk, try a different route. Go to a dog park and throw a ball in the park. Every extra step makes a difference. If you don't have a dog, walk a neighbor's pet! They will appreciate it.

Running

Suppose your body is in shape for a run. In that case, you will be surprised at how many physical and mental health benefits you will receive by decreasing the risk of heart disease to lowering stress levels. Take your pick, run around the block, or around the yard (if you want privacy).

Swimming

Have some fun and go for a swim. You will be giving your cardiovascular system a workout and strengthening many muscle groups. You can enjoy a fun - social outing while providing your body with aerobics and strength training into your exercise regime.

Tai Chi

The techniques used in Tai Chi are super relaxing and comes with its physical and mental benefits. The methods are enjoyed by many women over 50 as a low-impact activity. It's easy on muscles and can assist with flexibility and mobility. You can also exercise your memory skills as you learn the challenging sequences used in the art.

Pilates

In recent years, Pilates has become increasingly popular among the 50s crowd.
It's an excellent core body workout with more benefits in helping back and joint pain and improving posture.

Yoga

Go for it! The 50's generation enjoys yoga for maintaining or developing better flexibility and balance. Research suggests yoga can prevent heart disease, high blood pressure, and alleviate many aches and pains. It's also an excellent stress-buster too.

Get Dancing

If you get bored quickly and love to listen to music. Tune in to your favorite style of "get-up-and-go" music for motivation. Grab a broom and get to work. Dance through the chores. If you still have plenty of energy, go out for an evening of dancing!

Try Zumba

Get moving with Zumba. Some individuals have proclaimed they had spinal and hip arthritis and in size 16. After a few Zumba classes with the keto diet plan, the pounds dropped.

Treat Yourself

Obviously, you don't want to grab a loaded milkshake with a handful of M&M's since that would erase your genuine efforts of dropping the pounds. Instead, reward yourself as you reach your goals with a new pair of jeans, a manicure, or an early night date with a movie. Use one of your delicious recipes with your favorite keto beverage and relax.

Conclusion

I hope each chapter of the *Keto Diet - After 50* was informative and provided you with all of the tools you need to achieve your goals - whatever they may be.

The next step is to gather a day or two from your diet plan and make a list of the essentials. Be sure to use a list so you can stay on the 'ketogenic' path!

You can further your attempts to lose weight if you opt to use intermittent fasting methods using your new ketogenic recipes. Consider these as new ways to make your keto experience much easier to handle. These are two of the most popular ways:

Skip Meals

If you are interested in trying intermittent fasting, but you have an irregular schedule or are not sure if it is for you; then, try it and skip a meal or two now and then; maybe the intermittent type of fasting for you. Getting into a fasting routine is vital to see the maximum results, but that doesn't occasionally mean that fasting doesn't come with benefits.

What's more, once you have tried skipping a meal now and then, you can see for yourself just how easy it is, which in turn can lead to more positive changes down the line. With so many intermittent fasting options available, the odds are good that one fits your schedule, so give it a try. What have you got to lose (besides a few pounds)?

The 5:2 Technique

There are not that many statistics on this diet for women, but it is considered safe. For women, just restrict calories for two days each week by having two meals (250 calories each) or about ¼ of your regular calorie intake. Men can have 600 calories or 300 calories for 2 meals. The rule of thumb is based on men needing

2,400 calories and women 2,000 calories. Eat as you usually do for the remainder of the week using the ketogenic diet plan.

Soups are an excellent choice for your fasting days. These are several other examples:

- Tea

- Black coffee

- Plenty of water

- Generous portions of veggies

- Natural yogurt and berries

- Baked or boiled eggs

- Lean meat or grilled fish

- Cauliflower rice

You will soon find how easy it is to drop the pounds by following the ketogenic diet plan. Use your new 21-day meal plan. If there is a menu item you do not want that day, simply switch it using another ketogenic choice with the same carbs. You will figure it out, so grab a new recipe and get cooking!

As a person over 50, you may need to supplement your diet plan with a few essential supplements while on the ketogenic diet plan. These are mere suggestions, so you recognize the symptoms if you have lowered the level of some essential nutrients. You may experience headaches, fatigue, or nausea, which is sometimes called 'induction flu.' As you remove the carbs, your potassium and sodium (vital electrolytes) are also removed. Taking a supplement will help with these issues.

Potassium Supplement: You can become low in potassium in the short-term because of the vomiting and diarrhea that could go along with your early stages to the keto plan. Natural potassium can also be received through milk, whole grains, bananas, veggies, peas, and beans. It is recommended to take supplements because potassium also leaves your body with salt. As part of your well-prepared meal plan, you should receive 3000 to 4000 mg of potassium daily.

Sodium Supplements: You should receive at least one to two grams of extra sodium daily. Some of the pros accomplish this with bouillon cubes. Sea salt is a great option used in your diet plan. You should receive 3000 to 5000 mg of sodium daily.

Magnesium Supplement: For magnesium, 300-500 mg is an initial recommendation. Muscle cramps are your best indicator of depletion.

Keep in mind, these are optional suggestions; it's best to speak with your physician before you begin any diet plan to ensure your health is ready for the changes.

I would like to add a few extra tips on how you can maintain your ketogenic status daily. Skip the highest-ranking items to fill your plate using GPS, which includes grains + potatoes + sugar. These are your trouble spots for ketosis. Dining out can create issues for ketosis, but with your new-found knowledge, you can enjoy many selections at most dining establishments.

For starters, consider your breakfast options. Play it safe with eggs to start your day. Some counts will vary depending on how they are prepared. You will learn how to gauge them with each new recipe you add to your collection. For lunchtime, select from fish or chicken, including a delicious salad with chicken breast. Use caution for the dressing, but using plain vinegar or vinaigrette is tasteful and healthy. As dinner approaches, choose a fresh green veggie and a lean cut of meat for the main course. If you aren't ready for a steak, try a hamburger without a bun with a tempting broccoli entree.

Frequently visit restaurants that offer veggie platters, carving stations, salad bars, and healthy seafood options. For the condiments, consider using olive oil, butter, cheese, and sour cream - versus the sweeter options, which are loaded in carbs.

Wisely choose your drink options and include water, coffee (decaf is best), herbal or regular tea, and sparkling water. If you indulge in the spirits, consider having a shot with a bit of club soda.

Play a mind game and use a smaller plate for your buffet options. It will work since once your plate is full, you will stop and have less opportunity for a big scoop of mac and cheese. Take your time and enjoy a conversation with family and friends. Sip on your chosen beverage and enjoy your dining experience.

In conclusion, I hope you can spare a few minutes for a review on Amazon if you found this book useful in any way. It's always appreciated!